TRIGGER POINT
Self-Care Manual

TRIGGER POINT
Self-Care Manual

For Pain-Free Movement

Donna Finando, L.Ac., L.M.T.

Healing Arts Press
Rochester, Vermont

Healing Arts Press
One Park Street
Rochester, Vermont 05767
www.InnerTraditions.com

Healing Arts Press is a division of Inner Traditions International

Note to the reader: This book is intended as an informational guide. The remedies, approaches, and techniques described herein are meant to supplement, and not to be a substitute for, professional medical care or treatment. They should not be used to treat a serious ailment without prior consultation with a qualified health care professional.

Library of Congress Cataloging-in-Publication Data
Finando, Donna.
  Trigger point self-care manual for pain-free movement / Donna Finando.
    p. cm.
  ISBN 1-59477-080-8
  1. Myalgia—Treatment. 2. Acupuncture points. 3. Self-care, Health. I. Title.
  RC925.5.F56 2005
  616.7'4206—dc22

                                                        2005022481

Printed and bound in Canada at Transcontinental

10 9 8 7 6 5 4 3 2 1

Muscle art by Polan & Waski
Stretching illustrations by Jane Waski

Text design by Jon Desautels and layout by Priscilla Baker
This book was typeset in Bembo, with Warnock and Myriad used as display typefaces

To send correspondence to the author of this book, mail a first class letter to the author
c/o Inner Traditions • Bear & Company, One Park Street, Rochester, VT 05767, and we will forward
the communication.

Contents

Introduction

Movement is life. We all move. For some of us movement is a joy. For all of us movement should be pain free. As children we moved and played with abandon. Movement was natural, it was easy. In our teens and twenties we danced, we played ball. Maybe we injured ourselves a bit, but the injury healed by itself in a couple of days.

Now we're adults, and we still move. We're athletes. We're dancers. We're commuters, mothers, gardeners, accountants, truck drivers, lawyers, skiers, massage therapists, carpenters. Sometimes we move too much; sometimes we don't move enough. And at one time or another we move in ways that lead to pain. We jump too much or too high, we slip on the ice, we carry bags that are too heavy across an airport that is vast. We sit too much, we stare at a computer screen too long, we spend way too much time on that beautiful first day of spring cleaning up a winter-neglected garden.

Have you ever awakened a day or two following such exertion knowing something was wrong? There's a pain in the shoulder that really hurts. You aren't comfortable reaching behind your back to fasten your clothing and it hurts when you reach up for your seat belt. X-rays of your shoulder don't show anything conclusive. Your orthopedist says it's probably tendinitis or bursitis and prescribes anti-inflammatory medications.

A couple of weeks later the pain is no better. You aren't sleeping because you can't lie on your shoulder without distress. Now the pain is in the front and the back of your arm, maybe your chest, and it's going all the way down to your hand. At a follow-up visit with the doctor you get a prescription for physical therapy. The therapist shows you exercises to stretch and strengthen your shoulder. Maybe he applies some ultrasound to the area. It may help somewhat but the pain keeps coming back. In fact, you find that you are moving your arm less and less as time goes by. Your physical therapy prescription runs out but little has changed, and the doctor says the tests don't show anything significant—you'll have to live with the pain. In an effort to get down to the bottom of this problem you try chiropractic, but that doesn't really help. Maybe you try deep massage—it's painful but it provides some relief, yet the relief doesn't last very long. You haven't played tennis all summer because of the pain, and there's no way you can do any more gardening. You can feel despair building.

What is going on with your body?

→ The answer is this: Nobody has really checked your muscles. Only in the latter part of the last century has there been a growing awareness that the muscles themselves harbor knots that produce pain, weakness, restricted movement, and more. The tricky part about these knots, or *trigger points,* is that the pain is often felt far away from the muscle band that harbors the trigger point. Once trigger points develop in a muscle, a progressive snowball effect takes place if those trigger points are not reduced and eliminated—in compensating for one muscle's weakness another muscle becomes strained and develops trigger points, and so on through the myofascial chain. Left unattended, these muscular trigger points can last for years and lead to disabling pain, dysfunction, and disability that defies conventional medical diagnosis and treatment. Emotional distress inevitably follows as quality of life deteriorates. There is nothing more disturbing than weakness and pain that seems to have no resolution and no end.

→ Once they are identified, trigger points can be reduced. Doctors inject analgesics directly into the trigger points; acupuncturists use dry needling; massage therapists use manual pressure. This last technique for reducing and eliminating trigger points can be employed by everyone as a self-care approach, an approach that gives us power over our pain.

We all have the capability of finding and eliminating our own trigger points or trigger points in the muscles of those around us who are in pain. This is the key. It is what leads to having real power over our pain. All that is required is the desire to *feel* our own muscles, to *find* our trigger points and *work* on them, and then to modify the behaviors that produced the trigger points in the first place.

That's what this book is about. Using the information here you can take hold of your pain and do something that will help you to eliminate it. This approach teaches us that trigger points and the pain they cause are real. It demonstrates that our pain is truly muscular in nature and that there is something we can do to help ourselves. Using this manual, you can identify the muscles that are the sources of your pain. You can learn to feel the muscle, its taut bands and trigger points, and you can learn to use pressure and stretching techniques to reduce them. To maintain your health and strength, you will find several simple guidelines that you can easily incorporate into your daily life that will help you to reduce your chances of developing debilitating trigger points in the future.

Learning a new skill and body of knowledge takes some time and effort. However, in this case the personal rewards are great: freedom from pain, freedom from restriction, and a return to the activities that we love to do.

So how do you go about using what is offered in this manual to help you care for your own muscles?

1. Take a look at the pain pattern images at the beginning of each muscle section and identify those images that most closely resemble the location of your pain. Read through the information regarding the muscles that you've determined are the ones that might be causing your pain. Do the symptoms sound familiar? If they do, it's a good bet that you can start there; if not, read about some of the other muscles.

2. Look closely at the images of the muscle involved. Get a sense of which bones it attaches to and in which direction the muscle fibers go. It will help if you have a clear mental image of the area that you are going to touch, the placement of the muscle within that area, and the location of the trigger point within the muscle.

3. Feel your body to locate the bones that the muscle attaches to.

4. Feel your body to locate the muscle. Palpate the muscle with your fingertips. First palpate to identify where it attaches to the bones. Then palpate the muscle to identify taut bands it might contain. Palpate *across* the muscle fibers to locate taut bands. Taut bands can be as thick as small cables or as thin as guitar

strings, depending on the size of the muscle. They will be tender to the touch.

5. Isolate the taut band by palpating it *along the length* of its muscle fibers. As you palpate the taut band you'll be able to identify an area along its length that is more tender than adjacent areas. That's the trigger point.

6. Once you've found the trigger point, compress it using your fingers, a pencil eraser, a tennis ball, a squash ball, or any one of a number of different treatment aids available on the market today. (Appendix 2 directs you to helpful treatment tools.) You'll need to hold the compression for twenty to thirty seconds before beginning to feel the softening of the taut band under your fingers and the release of pain. This is something you'll have to repeat several times over the course of the day in order to obtain complete release.

7. Stretch the muscle after treatment. Read the directions carefully before stretching. Placing your body correctly is absolutely key to the proper stretching of the muscle. It doesn't take much to stretch most muscles; it does take attention to detail.

8. Use moist heat to complete the treatment. The use of a thermophore, hydrocollator, or wet heating pad is ideal. For the greatest benefit, position your body carefully in order to make sure that the muscle is relaxed when you use the heating pad.

9. Treat your muscles daily for several days in a row. Sometimes full release will take longer than that. It is almost never the case that only one muscle is involved and so your pain will probably change over the course of your treatment. If your pain doesn't change in a couple of days, check out a different muscle. You may not be treating the right muscle for your pain.

10. Remember that you are unwinding a Gordian knot, particularly if you've had this problem for a long time. Be patient; keep at it. You'll probably have to revisit this more than once. The more you learn about your own muscles, the more you'll be able to help yourself.

Take a few minutes to read the material presented in the introductory chapters to get a clear idea of what a trigger point is, how it develops, and what its associated symptoms are. The chapter on trigger points provides detailed palpation and treatment guidelines to provide a greater understanding of how to approach your pain.

A chapter on common musculoskeletal injuries differentiates types of injuries to make it easy for you to understand when you have trigger points and when there is an injury that requires medical intervention. Most serious injuries, such as fractures and joint locations, require medical attention; such injuries are also likely to lead to the development of trigger points in their associated muscles. Once an injury has healed, your muscles will need attention in order to complete the healing process.

And finally, read the concluding chapter on ways to maintain your general health: the best overall approach for injury prevention.

Remember: Movement is life. When we take care to ensure that our muscles remain soft and supple, not only can we own the power to help ourselves and take control of our pain, we can also offset some of the stiffness and weakness that inevitably creeps upon us as we enter our older years. When we take care of our muscles—when we take care of ourselves—we can remain vital and active, living life to its fullest and enjoying movement throughout the course of all our days.

CHAPTER 1

What Are Trigger Points and How Do I Treat Them?

Taken as a whole, the musculature is considered to be the largest single organ in the body. The system is comprised of approximately two hundred paired muscles (most muscles are mirrored on the right and left sides of the body) constituting 40 to 50 percent of the body's total weight. Muscles are utilized in all levels of body movement, from the gross to the miniscule, from the skeletal to the organic. They help to maintain our posture, they contain our internal organs, and through their movements they contribute to the maintenance of body heat.

When the muscles are impaired and cannot properly perform their role, the systems that they affect, contain, or control also become impaired. The implication is clear: When the muscles are dysfunctional there is ultimately an affect on the body as a whole. Yet the muscles are often the "neglected children" of conventional medical care. No medical specialty actually focuses on treatment of the muscles. They are frequently overlooked and may even be considered irrelevant in relationship to the overall healing of injuries.

When an injury occurs—a fracture, sprain, or dislocation—the concern for healing is rightly directed at the trauma, the break, the injured joint. As a result of this unilateral focus, innumerable people who have sustained an injury have healed, but they have healed only partially. They are returned to *almost* normal function but not *complete* function. Range of motion may be slightly limited, but it is limited. There may be a bit of stiffness, but there is stiffness.

That final bit of healing that has yet to occur is the healing of the musculature. The muscles are the agents of movement and joint stability. When a bone or joint is injured, the muscles that act on that joint must be given the attention that they require so that they may be returned to the length and strength that they owned prior to the injury.

Athletes know better than anyone that the little bit of muscular ache and stiffness not attended to may lead to chronic soreness and inflammation, which at the very least may reduce capability and force. Over time an even more severe injury may occur, when the proper practice of technique is sacrificed in an unconscious desire to avoid pain. Trainers and coaches know this pattern well. Their approach usually involves attending to the muscle through the use of rest and ice, parts one and two of the familiar RICE formula for care of musculoskeletal injuries, in order to avoid inflammation of the tissues. (The total RICE prescription is Rest, Ice, Compression, and Elevation.) Some trainers and coaches recommend massage and/or the use of moist heat or hot soaks in a tub to flush the tissues, in the hope of returning the muscles to their normal elastic state. Missing, however, is the awareness that muscles become injured in their own way.

Muscles are comprised of individual bands of muscle tissue lying parallel to one another. These bands work together when the muscle contracts. A muscular strain or trauma can lead to the restriction of one or more of these bands, resulting in what we call a "taut band." A trigger point will be located within the taut band. If you think of a muscle spasm as the contraction of a whole muscle, it follows that a taut band is like a microspasm, a "spasm" of an individual band of the muscle. The muscular dysfunction caused by the taut band will remain until the taut band is released.

Muscles are wonderful structures. They are supple, elastic, resilient, and powerful. You know when they are healthy because your movement is fluid, easy, unrestricted. You bend with ease. Standing, reaching, and twisting take place without a second thought. Joints move freely without a hint of discomfort or limitation. When your muscles are healthy you don't think about them, except for the joy and exhilaration that movement brings. When you touch them they're soft. You can easily feel the underlying structures, the bones that lie beneath them. They aren't tender to the touch; they don't hurt.

When a muscle develops taut bands and trigger points it becomes constricted. It feels tight to the touch. It loses its elasticity and suppleness. If it remains constricted over time there might be a reduction of blood supply to the muscle, making it more fibrous and less elastic. You might well experience the steady, deep, dull, aching pain or tenderness associated with trigger points in the muscles, a condition that has been termed a myofascial pain syndrome. Each trigger point produces a predictable pain pattern that is reproducible when the trigger point is compressed.* Interestingly enough, the pain frequently is not located at the site of the muscular trigger point. Pain resulting from a trigger point, what is known as referred pain, is felt at a distance from the trigger point. This is important to remember because it means that a person can look at an image of a pain pattern to find out which muscle is involved in producing that pain.

So how does a muscle develop trigger points? It usually begins with some form of mechanical abuse or overload. Active people between the ages of thirty and fifty are most at risk for developing trigger points and suffering with the resulting myofascial pain. However, it doesn't take an athletic endeavor to be on the receiving end of trigger point pain. Trigger points can develop from an unexpected missed step, landing the wrong way from a jump, sleeping in the wrong position, reaching too far to return a tennis serve, using a poorly positioned computer, playing too much softball after taking the winter off, gardening with abandon on the first warm day of spring, carrying a huge box filled with books up stairs, or sitting at your desk or on a plane for an extended period of time. The list of causes for trigger point activation is endless because the possibilities for movement are endless.

Mechanical abuse of the muscle can occur as a result of either *overuse* or *overload*.

Overuse of a muscle often takes place when the muscle is put to work over and over again, performing the same action in the same way. Going out to practice your backhand in tennis and hitting one hundred balls is a good example of overuse. The next day your elbow is sore and you believe you may have developed tennis elbow. What's happened is that the forearm muscles have been taken through the same action, over and over again, far in excess of what they normally do. They have become shortened, developed taut bands and trigger points. The trigger points have referred pain to the elbow.

---

*David G. Simons, Janet G. Travell, and Lois S. Simons, *Travell and Simons': Myofascial Pain and Dysfunction, The Trigger Point Manual*, vol. 1, 2nd ed. (Baltimore: Williams and Wilkins, 1999), 5, 6.

Something that I have taken to calling "trainer-induced injuries" is an example of muscle *overload*. A weight trainer has you doing quadriceps extensions. You've already done three sets of twelve repetitions. Your trainer encourages: "Just one more rep, one more." Your body is crying out to stop because your muscles are fatigued and you simply cannot imagine being able to do one more rep. Yet you do it. The following day when you get out of bed you find that you can't stand straight because your thighs are terribly sore, beyond the normal charley horse that you've experienced before. The pain lasts for days; it's unrelenting and it markedly affects your ability to walk, climb stairs, and sit down. An overloaded muscle is one that is made to exert more force than the muscle is physically capable of.

Overloading a muscle can take place in one of three ways. In our example here, the injury was in response to a *repetitive overload*.

Acute overload is another way in which a muscle can be injured. In acute overload you suddenly and often unexpectedly place way too much force on the muscle. Imagine this scenario. A martial artist is demonstrating a throw with an inexperienced student. As he takes hold of the student and tries to bring him to the ground, the student holds on for dear life. This results in an acute overload to the back muscles of the martial artist, who unexpectedly has to deal with a 175-pound weight on his back.

A *sustained overload* might be experienced when you find that you have to carry the weight of a heavy box of books up not one flight of stairs, as expected, but up three or four flights. In addition to overuse and overload, *direct trauma*, trauma that occurs by impact, such as by getting tackled in a football game, can be the source of muscular trigger points, as can the trauma that might result from a fall or automobile accident. *Chilling* of the muscle can cause trigger points to develop as well.

There are different types of trigger points. *Latent trigger points* represent the vast majority of trigger points present in the musculature. Everyone has them. Latent trigger points develop as the result of postural habits, strains, overuse, chronic disease, and recurrent emotional and physical patterns of behavior. Latent trigger points produce stiffness and weakness in the affected muscles and restrict full range of motion of the joints that the affected muscles act on. Latent trigger points will not release without direct release techniques and they may easily persist for years.

The chronic tightness in the upper shoulders that just about everybody experiences is an example of latent trigger points in the upper trapezius muscle. You might feel muscle tightness or restriction when you try to stretch your upper shoulder by aiming your ear toward your shoulder. When you touch the center of the rounded part of your upper shoulder and press into it, in all likelihood you will feel a tender "knot" there. That's your trigger point. It developed because of the way you hold your arms and shoulders or because of the way you use your shoulder to talk on the phone.

Through a bit of overuse or an unexpected overload, that latent trigger point can become an active trigger point. An *active trigger point* in a muscle produces a predictable referred pain pattern that is specific to that muscle. Each muscle has its own referred pain pattern. When that latent trigger point in your upper trapezius becomes active, in addition to the stiffness, weakness, and reduced range of motion you will begin to feel a deep, aching pain that might go right up to your skull behind your ear. The muscle might be so locked up and the trigger point so irritable that the pain might go around your ear into your temple. There may have been a specific incident that produced the active trigger point, or the onset may have taken place gradually, over a period of time. The muscles located within the pain pattern may be tender to the touch. This tenderness will dissipate after the trigger point has been reduced.

Pain from active trigger points varies in intensity during the course of the day. Pain will increase with use of the muscle, during stretching of the muscle, upon direct pressure to the trigger point, with prolonged shortening or repetitive contraction of the muscle, in cold or damp weather, and in the company of viral infections and stress. Conversely, symptoms will decrease after short periods of rest and with slow, passive stretching of the muscle, particularly during the application of moist heat to the muscle.

We've said that trigger points are *directly* activated through overuse, overload, direct trauma, and chilling. But trigger points can be *indirectly* activated as well. Disease of the internal organs, particularly the heart, gall bladder, kidneys, and stomach, can produce trigger points in their associated musculature. Joint disease or dysfunction, such as arthritis, puts an overload strain on the surrounding musculature, and can therefore be the source of trigger points in those muscles.

Immobilizing the muscle or keeping the muscle in a shortened position for an extended period of time can produce trigger points. Emotional distress can lead to trigger points as well.

When a muscle lies within the pain pattern produced by other active trigger points, trigger points can develop in that muscle as well. We call these *satellite* trigger points.

Generally, the degree of conditioning of the muscle is the factor that most defines whether a latent trigger point will become active. Strongly conditioned muscles are less susceptible to trigger point activation than poorly conditioned muscles. Active trigger points will frequently return to latency with sufficient rest; however, trigger points will not be fully reduced without direct treatment. People frequently report that the pain keeps coming back, sometimes over periods of years, and this is the reason why.

How are trigger points treated? First, the trigger point must be located within the muscle. This is done by *palpating,* feeling the muscle with your fingers. Once the trigger point is located, the medical professional might use an analgesic or anesthetic injection; an acupuncturist may use acupuncture needles; a physical therapist might use modalities such as ultrasound or electrical stimulation, possibly combined with muscle-energy technique or a technique called post-isometric relaxation.

The manual or massage therapist will use compression, applying direct pressure to the trigger point. This is a technique that we can all use for self-care. The key is in finding the trigger point. Many trigger points are located in predictable locations; however, owing to physical differences, trigger points can be located in any muscle and in any location within a muscle.

In their most healthy state your muscles are elastic and supple; touching them shouldn't hurt at all. But if the inside of your knee was painful and your knee was buckling, the muscle on the inside of your thigh close to your knee wouldn't feel so supple. Moving your hands and fingers over that muscle you would recognize that, rather than a ball of pliable dough the muscle might feel as though there were taut, stringy bands in it. It is within those taut bands that you will find the trigger points.

You will have to palpate your muscles to get a sense of the difference between soft, pliable muscles and muscles that contain taut bands. This likely sounds more difficult than it is. Just relax and bring your curiosity into your hands and try to "see" with your fingers. You will be delighted by what you will be able to feel.

When you palpate your muscle you will need to feel it throughout its length. Take a moment right now to feel your body—place your fingers and the palm of your hand on the middle of your thigh. Imagine that your thigh muscle, quadriceps femoris, is clay that you are molding or dough that you are kneading. Press into your thigh with your entire hand: your palm, fingers, and fingertips. Quadriceps femoris runs along the length of your thigh, from your hip to your knee. Try to feel for a taut band by moving your hand crosswise over the muscle. Feel *across* the length of the muscle, not *along* its length. As you feel across the length of the muscle you'll be able to identify a taut band; it will feel tender to the touch. In a muscle as large as quadriceps femoris the taut band might feel as broad as a thin cable; in smaller muscles taut bands can feel as thin as guitar strings.

Once you've found a taut band, keep your fingers on it. Try to isolate it from the surrounding musculature. Follow it through its length and you will come to an area that is very tender, more tender than any other area in the band. You might even note that when you apply pressure directly to that spot there is an involuntary twitch of the muscle. This is what Travell calls a "twitch response."★ This most tender spot is the trigger point.

Once you've found the trigger point, press into it—use your finger, a pencil eraser, a tennis ball, a squash ball, or one of the many products currently on the market that are designed to apply pressure to trigger points. (See appendix 2 for information on such products.) Any of these will allow you to compress the trigger point. Hold the compression for twenty to thirty seconds. With a moderate amount of pressure, the point will hurt. Note that with trigger point release more is not necessarily better. Press just enough to feel the tightness of the band and the soreness of the trigger point and then keep your pressure at that level. Don't press into it any harder.

While you are maintaining that pressure for a few moments you will feel two wonderful things—the tenderness underneath your fingers will start to reduce and the tightness under your fingers will begin to let go—you will feel the release of the muscle. As the muscle releases you can increase your pressure just a bit more to "follow" it with your fingers. Over the course of several sessions where

★Simons, Travell, and Simons, *The Trigger Point Manual*, vol. 1, 34.

you work on the muscle in this way you will begin to notice that the pain in your knee has been reduced, and at some point you will note that your knee hasn't buckled for a while.

After working on the muscle it's important to stretch and then apply moist heat. Stretching lengthens the muscle, helping it to return to its normal suppleness and resting length. With each muscle description in this book I've provided a stretch or stretches to specifically target that muscle. These stretches were designed to work individual muscles, not large muscle groups. When you stretch it's very important to place your body correctly in order to lengthen the specific muscle that you're targeting. You'll know you're in the right position as soon as you begin stretching—you won't have to stretch very far to feel it in the muscle. It's important to do the stretches frequently throughout the course of the day. A briefly held stretch done six or seven times a day is far more useful than holding a stretch for a long time only once a day. You are reeducating the muscle to return to its normal resting length—as in any training regimen, repetition is key.

The combination of stretching and breathing is both wonderful for your muscles and an essential component to the healing process. Your muscles will naturally relax when you exhale. With each exhale let your body release into the stretch.

The application of moist heat completes the treatment by bringing blood and fluids to the muscle, increasing circulation to the area and allowing the muscle to return to its normal, healthy metabolic state. It will also help relieve some muscle soreness that might result from your trigger point release work. Moist heat can be applied in the form of a wet heating pad, a thermophore, or a hydrocollator applied directly to the muscle for twenty minutes once or twice a day.

Care should be taken to put your body in a position in which the moist heat can be applied directly to the *relaxed* muscle, a muscle that isn't in use. For example, if you want to apply a moist heating pad to the muscles at your low back, it is best done while you are lying on your belly with a pillow placed under your ankles. In this position your low back muscles are relaxed. If you try to apply moist heat to these muscles while you're in a seated position, your back muscles will be working to keep your body erect. The moist heat will be far less effective. A hot bath or warm shower can be helpful, but they aren't as useful as applying a moist heating pad directly to the area.

Understanding what trigger points are, identifying trigger points in your musculature, treating those points, stretching the muscles involved, and applying moist heat: this is your recipe for self-treatment. And it is this recipe that can lead you to a pain-free, active life.

CHAPTER 2

Common Musculoskeletal Injuries and Trigger Points

Each of us who has participated in a sport or physical art understands how readily injuries can occur, particularly as we move through our teens and twenties into our middle years. Up until quite recently, most of the information that has been disseminated regarding injuries has been with respect to those very serious injuries that occur to the musculoskeletal system and that have a way of preventing us from practicing our sport for an extended period of time. These injuries affect the bones, the ligaments (which attach bones to bones), the tendons (which attach muscles to bones), and the muscles themselves. What these injuries have in common is their effect on the musculature.

When a bone, joint, or ligament is injured the muscles that surround the area undergo changes that often lead to trigger point development. This can result from the trauma that caused the injury, from immobilization that healing of the injury required, or from weakness that resulted from lack of use during healing. Once the bone or joint is healed, it is essential for the restrictions within the musculature to be addressed through trigger point release.

Physical therapy for muscle strengthening is often prescribed subsequent to the healing of an injury. Why is it insufficient or ineffective so much of the time? Because the muscle cannot be strengthened before any taut bands and trigger points within the muscle have been released, returning the muscle to its normal resting length. That's where you come in. Understand that when you have a skeletal injury the bones need to heal properly. Once they are healed, the muscles acting on those bones need to be worked on for complete release in order for true healing to take place.

Let's look at the characteristics of the various types of injuries.

A crack or break in a bone is a *fracture*. Fractures are generally accompanied by swelling, extreme pain, and tenderness in the injured area. There is generally a change in appearance of the injured part that may include protruding bone or blood under the skin. The extremity—the arm, leg, or finger—may be bent out of shape. A fracture can occur to any bone. Some fractures require surgical intervention in order to stabilize the bone; others require splinting or casting in order to maintain the proper position of the bones until healing begins. It is recommended that medical care be obtained as quickly as possible in the event of a fracture.

The muscles that act on the region of the fracture will be affected by a fracture as well. Both the trauma to the body part and the subsequent immobilization necessary for healing will impact the muscles. Trigger points develop from both trauma and immobilization. Therefore, after the bone has healed you should work on the musculature to identify and reduce areas of restriction within the muscles. This will have the dual effect of contributing to the complete recovery of the area and precluding the potential of muscular difficulties.

A *stress fracture* or *fatigue fracture* is a fracture that occurs at a microscopic level. A stress fracture often occurs as a result of repetitive overuse or with an increase in activity. This kind of fracture may signal the presence of osteoporosis. Pain resulting from a stress fracture may develop slowly, over time. It may begin with a diffuse, dull ache and progress to a localized area of concentrated pain, intensified by impact. A stress fracture may not show up on x-ray or other studies until one to two weeks after its occurrence, when bone healing has begun. Because the fracture is generally stable and does not require splinting or casting, treatment is often limited to the restriction of activity. Stress fractures commonly occur at the hip, at either of the long bones of the lower leg (the tibia and the fibula), and at the metatarsal bones of the foot.

Repeated stresses, such as prolonged standing, running, jogging, jumping, dancing, or walking, are often the source of stress fractures. Symptoms usually include mild swelling, discoloration of the area, tenderness to the touch, warmth at the site of the fracture, and pain that is alleviated by rest. Treatment of a stress fracture can include rest, ice, and elevation of the affected body part.

The activities that cause a stress fracture also cause trigger points in the musculature, and complete healing requires care of that musculature. During the time required for healing the stress fracture, work on the muscles that act on that body part in order to reduce taut bands and trigger points. Those muscles include the muscles of the low back, buttocks, thighs, and lower legs. The increased circulation that results from the release of the musculature will have the added benefit of decreasing healing time and allowing you to return to your activities sooner rather than later.

A *joint dislocation* is a disruption of the normal relationship between the bones that form a joint. The dislocation may be momentary and self-correcting; however, depending on its severity the injury might require medical attention in order to return the bones to their normal positions. Common sites of dislocations are the shoulder, wrist, hand, finger, hip, knee, ankle, and jaw. Dislocations affect the ligaments that hold the bones in place and also affects the surrounding muscles, tendons, nerves, and blood vessels. Symptoms accompanying a dislocation may include severe pain at the time of the occurrence, visible deformity of the body part, loss of function of the joint, tenderness, swelling, bruising, and possibly numbness. Immediate first aid includes the application of RICE—rest, ice, compression, and elevation—particularly within the first twenty-four hours and then as prescribed by your physician.

It's important to remember that, with a dislocation, the muscles that act on the affected joint will also be affected by the dislocation and will require treatment in order to heal completely. They will have suffered an acute strain and will likely develop taut bands and trigger points. Once the swelling and tenderness of the area immediately surrounding the joint has healed, work on the muscles that act on the joint. They are each likely to have developed restrictions, taut bands, and trigger points. This will have the dual effect of contributing to the complete recovery of the area and precluding potential muscular difficulties.

A *sprain* is the violent overstretching of one or more ligaments surrounding a joint; when the ligament is overstretched it may give way at its weakest point, either where it attaches to the bone or within the ligament itself. Sprain is accompanied by severe pain at the time of injury, a feeling of popping or tearing at the joint site, tenderness at the injury site, swelling, and bruising. Ligaments have an extremely limited blood supply; their healing time may therefore be as long as the healing of a fracture. With a sprain it is extremely important to allow adequate time for rest and healing prior to the return of activity. Doing so will avert the possibility of joint instability and repeated, increasingly severe, sprains. The ankle and the knee are common sites for ligament tearing.

Sprains are graded as mild, moderate, and severe.

- A mild (grade I) sprain involves the tearing of some ligament fibers. There is no loss of function. The average healing time is two to six weeks.
- A moderate (grade II) sprain involves the rupture of a portion of a ligament. There is some loss of function. The average healing time is between six and eight weeks. Healing may require immobilization of the joint.
- A severe (grade III) sprain is the complete rupture of the ligament or a complete separation of the ligament from the bone. There is total loss of function. A severe sprain requires surgical repair followed by immobilization. The average healing time is eight weeks to ten months.

Immediate first aid for a sprain is the application of RICE—rest, ice, compression, and elevation—particularly within the first twenty-four hours. Medical evaluation will determine the extent of the sprain and appropriate follow-up therapy.

It's important to remember that the muscles that act on the affected joint will also be impacted by the sprain and will require treatment in order to heal completely. It is likely that they will develop taut bands and trigger points in response to the injury. While the joint is healing from the sprain, identify the muscles that act on the joint and work on their taut bands and trigger points. This will contribute to the complete recovery of the area, and it may preclude the possibility of future muscular difficulties.

Bursitis is an inflammation of a bursa, the fluid-filled sac that lies between adjacent structures, providing cushioning and reducing friction between them. The purpose of a bursa is to allow one structure to glide freely over another. Bursae lie between the skin and bony protrusions such as the elbow or the kneecap; between tendons and ligaments; and between tendons, ligaments, and bones. Bursitis develops slowly over time; it is associated with chronic overuse of an area and with trauma, arthritis, or infection. Without appropriate treatment bursitis may develop into a recurring problem.

Symptoms associated with bursitis include pain that is worse during the night and in the morning upon rising. Pain may be severe until the area is moved, at which point pain recedes. Pain may return after a period of moderate movement or exercise. Pain is generally located over the site of the bursa. It is accompanied by tenderness, swelling, limitation of motion of the affected region, and (if the inflammation is severe) redness and fever. Commonly affected sites include the shoulder, elbow, knee, and hip. Treatment of bursitis includes the use of RICE—rest, ice, compression, and elevation. However, your physician can make a precise diagnosis and prescribe treatment appropriate to your needs.

Bursitis can be differentiated from pain caused by trigger points in that bursitis is accompanied by swelling in the region of pain, whereas pain caused by trigger points is not. However, because chronic overuse is associated with the onset of bursitis, it is possible that the musculature that acts on the affected joint may contain taut bands and trigger points. Identifying taut bands and reducing trigger points will contribute to the healing process by increasing circulation to the area and reducing muscular restrictions that may contribute to friction in and around the joint.

Tendinitis is an inflammation of a tendon, the structure that attaches muscle to bone. Tendinitis will often develop as a result of chronic overuse, repetitive action, engaging in activity without stretching and warming up sufficiently, or stretching the tendon beyond its normal capabilities; or, in the case of occasional sports participants (so-called weekend warriors), overdoing activity with insufficient muscular conditioning. Symptoms associated with tendinitis include pain and tenderness along the tendon—usually close to the affected joint—a generalized ache in the region, and swelling. Pain is worse with movement and may be worse at night. Heat and redness may be present over the site of the tendon. Common sites for tendinitis are the elbow, shoulder, knee, and ankle. Elbow tendinitis, known in the medical lexicon as *epicondylitis,* is referred to as "tennis elbow." When it occurs on the inside of the elbow it is called *medial epicondylitis,* and when it occurs at the outside of the elbow it is *lateral epicondylitis.* Tendinitis of the knee, known as patellar/quadriceps tendinitis or "jumper's knee," is an inflammation of the tendon that attaches the quadriceps femoris muscle to the lower leg. Achilles tendinitis is tendinitis of the Achilles tendon, the tendon that attaches the calf muscle to the back of the heel. Self-care includes the application of ice, particularly after engaging in a sports activity.

The referred pain from trigger points is often misdiagnosed as tendinitis. The difference between the two is that, with tendinitis, swelling and possibly heat and/or redness are present in addition to tenderness at the site. When trigger points are the source of pain there is no swelling, heat, or redness. However, in both cases there may be taut bands in the musculature that act on the involved joint. That being the case, it is essential to work on the muscles that act on the joint: on the forearm muscles in the case of tennis elbow, the quadriceps femoris in the case of jumper's knee, the gastrocnemius and soleus in the case Achilles tendinitis, and the biceps brachii and rotator cuff muscles in the case of tendinitis of the shoulder.

A *strain* is an injury to the muscles or to the tendons (which attach muscle to bone). A strain is often caused by chronic overuse of a muscle or prolonged or repetitive action. Overloading a muscle or sustaining trauma to an area causes acute strains. Strains are generally accompanied by pain while moving or stretching the body part, muscle spasm in surrounding areas, swelling over the site, loss of strength, and—in a severe strain—crepitus, a grating or crackling sound when the area is compressed.

Strains are graded as mild, moderate, or severe.

• A mild (grade I) strain is known as a "pulled muscle." The muscle or the fibers of the muscle tendon do not tear and strength is not diminished. A mild strain requires an average of two to ten days' healing time.
• A moderate (grade II) strain, a "torn muscle," involves the tearing of fibers in a muscle, in its tendon, or at the attachment of the muscle to the bone. Strength is somewhat diminished. A moderate strain requires ten days to six weeks' healing time.
• A severe (grade III) strain involves a rupture of the muscle-tendon-bone attachment with separation of fibers. Strength is considerably diminished and crepitus, a grating or crackling sound, is felt and heard when the area is pressed with the finger. A severe strain requires surgical repair and requires six to ten weeks' healing time.

Immediate first aid for a strain is the application of RICE—rest, ice, compression, and elevation—particularly within the first twenty-four hours. Medical evaluation will determine the extent of the strain and appropriate follow-up therapy.

It's important to remember that muscle strains are one of the primary causes of the development of taut bands and trigger points in muscles. Eliminating taut bands and reducing trigger points precludes the possibility of future muscular difficulties. Identify the muscles that are involved and locate their taut bands and trigger points; their release will increase circulation and will contribute to the complete recovery of the area. Treatment, allowing adequate healing time before returning to your normal sports activities, warming up prior to exercise, and conditioning the musculature will help to prevent further muscle strains.

A *spasm,* or *cramp,* is a sudden and involuntary contraction of a muscle. This frequently painful contraction produces a hard, bulging muscle. The causes of muscle spasms are varied: muscle fatigue brought on by overworking the muscle or staying in one position for too long; dehydration; insufficient stretching and warming up prior to engaging in an activity; imbalances of calcium, magnesium, or potassium; pregnancy; poor circulation; diabetes; alcoholism; kidney disease; and side effects of medications. "Splinting spasms" may occur as a mechanism that serves to inhibit movement in order to protect an injured or unstable region of the body. Calf cramps often occur at night; they are referred to as "nocturnal calf cramps." A cramp is usually temporary and can be relieved with slow stretching, the application of moist heat or ice, and gentle massage to the area. Medical evaluation is advised if cramps are severe, prolonged, or recurrent.

Muscular pain and soreness due to muscle spasm usually diminishes with the release of the spasm. Some residual soreness may remain for a brief period of time. Taut bands and trigger points generally do not develop as a result of a spasm or cramp.

Delayed onset muscle soreness (DOMS) is familiar to many of us. It commonly occurs after a workout or exercise, particularly if you aren't used to working out, if you are using different muscles than you are accustomed to, or if you are using your muscles differently than usual. Muscle stiffness, weakness, or soreness starts between eight and twenty-four hours following exercise; it peaks between twenty-four and seventy-two hours and it usually dissipates within three to seven days. *Delayed onset muscle soreness* occurs with overloading the muscle through stretch, resistance, or excessive activity. Activities that require a muscle to contract while lengthening seem to cause the greatest soreness. The standard biceps curl is an example of such a movement. The exertion that is made while flexing the muscle isn't the source of the soreness; it's the exertion while slowly straightening the arm that produces the overload. When you're straightening the arm the biceps muscle is exerting force while lengthening. It is generally thought that microscopic muscle tearing and associated tissue swelling within the muscle is the source of the soreness. The degree of muscle damage is related to the intensity of soreness present and the speed with which the soreness is initially felt.

Delayed onset muscle soreness is unaffected by the application of heat and ice and anti-inflammatory medications. Sometimes light activity, stretching, and gentle massage help to reduce the pain, probably due to the increased circulation to the musculature.

Taut bands and trigger points do not generally develop subsequent to delayed onset muscle soreness.

Musculoskeletal injury is an all-too-common occurrence for athletes and dancers. Self-treatment is useful and has its place within the context of general care. However, it is important to seek professional help in these circumstances:

- when numbness, tingling, or shooting pain is present
- when a limb or region becomes cold or turns white or blue
- when swelling, heat, redness, and fever are unresponsive to first aid measures within forty-eight hours
- when pain persists for more than seven to ten days
- when other areas begin to hurt due to compensation for an injured area
- when oral medications are needed for pain relief for more than two to three days
- when pain interrupts or disrupts your sleep for more than one or two nights
- when you are unable to bear your own weight

It has become increasingly clear that we have to take personal responsibility for our health and well-being. We have to be clear about when it is important to seek medical attention. We have to be equally clear when conventional medical treatment stops short of providing us with the means with which to completely heal. Understanding the nature of physical injury and what is required for the healing of that injury is part of taking on that responsibility. This book will help you in that endeavor.

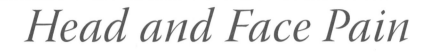

Head and Face Pain

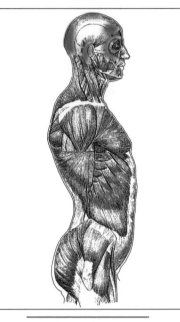

Pain pattern: Sternocleidomastoid

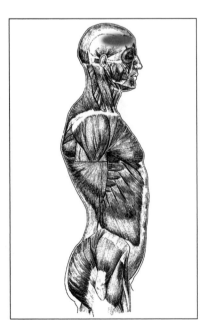

Semispinalis capitis

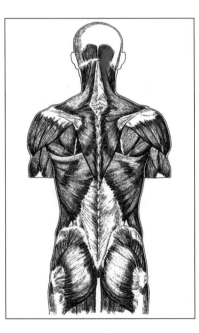

Semispinalis cervicis

Pain pattern: Posterior cervicals

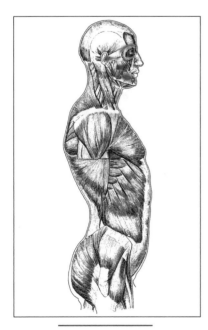

Pain pattern: Splenius capitis

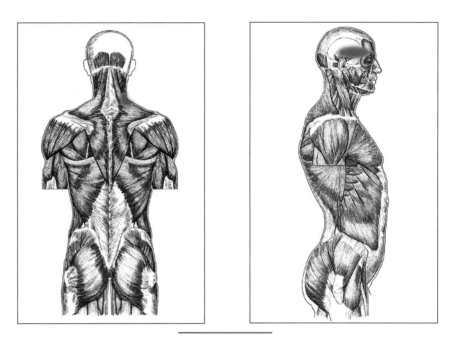

Pain pattern: Splenius cervicis

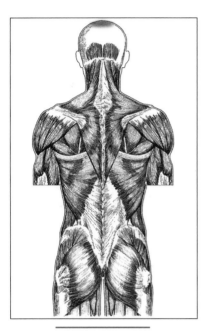

Pain pattern: Masseter

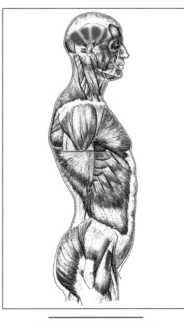

Pain pattern: Temporalis

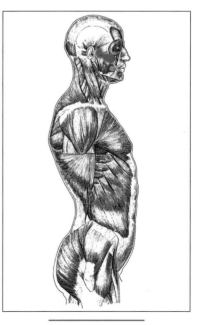

Pain pattern: Pterygoids

Eight cranial bones and fourteen facial bones form the structure of the skull. Suspended from the skull is the head's only moveable bone, the mandible, known colloquially as the jawbone. Upon the bones of the skull lie the fifteen muscles through which we express most of our emotions, and the four muscles that move the lower jaw, allowing us to bite, grind, and chew food.

For most of us the face is the focal point of our sense of self. Rather than feeling our sense of self in the belly, chest, legs, or back, we identify ourselves with and in our face and head. This is one of the primary reasons that headache and facial pain can be so debilitating; pain in this region intrudes on our ability to function in ways that other bodily aches and pains do not. It interferes with our ability to think, to concentrate, and sometimes to see clearly. You can't get away from head or face pain.

Head and facial pain often occurs as a function of injury or strain of the neck muscles, particularly when the head is held in extension (when it is dropped back slightly). Whiplash is often the source of injury, whether the whiplash has taken place as a result of an automobile accident or a fall. A fall secondary to being tackled from behind is the perfect example. Tackled from behind, the head flies backward before it is thrust forward. This is the recipe for sternocleidomastoid (SCM) injury—the trademark whiplash.

Straining the neck while holding it in extension is another source of injury. Think about it—the upper body bent forward over bent legs, head up, chin jutting forward. This head posture is common in football, tennis and other racket sports, in swimming the breaststroke, and in bicycling. Sitting in the front rows of a theater or painting your ceiling will place your head and neck in the same position. Consider what this position is doing to the neck muscles—the muscles in the front of the neck are lengthened and the muscles in the back of the neck are shortened. This posture inevitably leads to weakness of the neck musculature and the development of trigger points.

Keeping the head and neck bent forward in flexion for extended periods of time can be equally problematic. Lying in bed with your chin on your chest as you read a book or watch television is a prescription for restriction in the neck muscles. That muscular restriction may cause facial pain resembling sinus headache as well as phenomena that are generally considered to be completely unrelated to the musculature such as dizziness, imbalance, and tearing of the eye. Using a computer monitor that is positioned below your line of sight can do the same thing.

Overuse or improper use of the muscles that are involved in chewing—the temporalis, masseter, and the pterygoids—will often lead to trigger points and resultant facial pain. Because of its location and associated symptoms, pain from trigger points in the head, neck, and facial muscles is often diagnosed as TMJ syndrome, a dysfunction of the temporomandibular joint. The temporomandibular joint connects your jawbone to your skull. The joint is located just in front of your ear. Place your index finger on the side of your face in front of the center of your ear, then open and close your mouth; you will feel the movement of the TMJ. You can also place your finger inside your ear and feel the movement of the joint as you open and close your mouth. Clenching a mouth guard or clenching onto a snorkel or regulator while diving produces overuse or improper use of those muscles, as will the automatic clenching of the teeth when lifting heavy weights, regardless of whether those weights are physical or emotional. Direct trauma to the jaw or habitually holding the head in a head-forward posture also places strain on these muscles and can lead to jaw dysfunction.

If you have head or facial pain, consider the symptoms that are associated with each of these muscles. Once you've identified the muscles that are involved, find and release their trigger points. But don't stop there. Check out the rest of the muscles in this section—see if there are taut bands in those muscles as well. It's highly likely that there will be. Release them all and stretch them all. You'll be glad you did.

Sternocleidomastoid

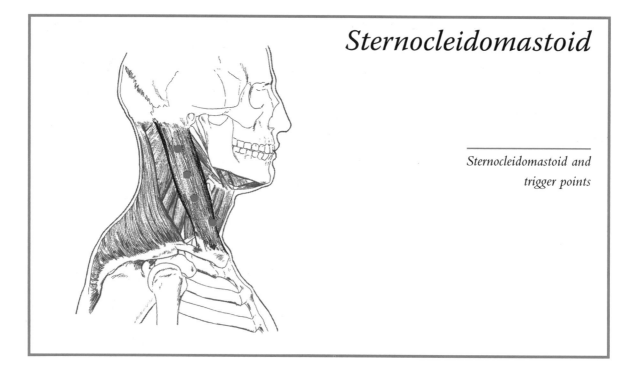

*Sternocleidomastoid and
trigger points*

THE STERNOCLEIDOMASTOID MUSCLE, the SCM, is a large muscle that lies on the side and front of the neck. Its name describes where its attachments are—on the breastbone or sternum *(sterno)*, the collarbone or clavicle *(cleido)*, and the bump on the base of your skull behind your ear, the mastoid process *(mastoid)*. The SCM acts in many different ways. When only one SCM is working, it turns and tilts your head to one side. When both muscles are working at the same time, the SCM flexes your neck, allowing your chin to drop down toward your chest, and it controls the backward motion of your head. Working with the trapezius, the SCM helps to stabilize the position of the head when your jaw moves, which is every time you speak or chew. Think about how hard this muscle has to work—the human head weighs as much as eight pounds!

Trigger points often develop in the SCM as a result of a whiplash injury. A whiplash is the forceful, unexpected, uncontrolled forward-then-backward motion of the head. Auto accidents are a well-known cause of whiplash injuries. So are falls, something that every athlete is at risk for. Keeping the head down for extended periods of time as well as extending it back for periods of time can create overuse injuries, another source of trigger points. Think of the position of the tennis player who is practicing receiving serves—the forward bend at the waist with head up is exactly one to strain the SCM. It is a familiar position for football players and skiers. Wrestlers practicing "bridges" are practically looking for trigger points in those positions!

Trigger points in the SCM don't refer pain to the neck at all. The most common symptom of trigger points in the SCM is pain in the forehead, most of the time on the same side as the involved muscle; when trigger points are severe, pain can be felt across the entire forehead. Pain might also be experienced deep in the ear. Trigger points can produce pain in the cheek and temple and around the eye. There can be pain and scalp tenderness right at the top of your head. Symptoms unrelated to pain include dizziness and lack of balance, tearing and redness of your eye, visual disturbances, and increased mucus production in the sinuses. You might also develop a dry cough.

To identify the sternocleidomastoid, look in a mirror and turn your head slightly toward your left side, then tilt your right ear toward your right shoulder; you'll see the bulge of the SCM on your right as it contracts to perform this action. You can easily grasp the muscle between your thumb and fingers and follow its course from the collarbone all the way up to the base of the skull.

Once you're clear on where the muscle is, relax your neck and head and allow the muscle to relax. Grasp the muscle using a pincer technique, using both your thumb and your fingers. Massage the muscle through its length, feeling for tender spots. You can locate trigger points on both sides of the SCM. Once you've found a sore spot, hold it and massage: direct pressure followed by tiny circles directly on the trigger point works nicely. Leave the trigger point for a few seconds and then return to it.

Working on the SCM can be quite painful. Don't live by the "no pain, no gain" formula with trigger points in this muscle. Pain that is bearable will produce results; pain that is unbearable will produce an irritated SCM.

Follow up working on the muscle with stretches.

1. Bend your head and neck backward, rotating the face to one side. The SCM on the opposite side will receive the stretch.
2. Turn your head to one side. When your head is turned all the way, tilt the chin toward the shoulder. The SCM on the side to which you have turned will receive the stretch.

Because the SCM is activated when you breathe up into your chest, it's important to train yourself to breathe deeply into your lower abdomen. See page 173 for specifics on how to do this.

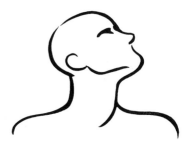

Stretch 1: Sternocleidomastoid, clavicular head

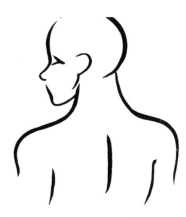

Stretch 2: Sternocleidomastoid, sternal head

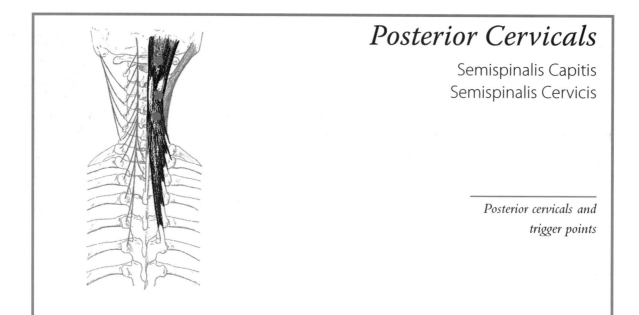

Posterior Cervicals

Semispinalis Capitis
Semispinalis Cervicis

Posterior cervicals and
trigger points

THE POSTERIOR CERVICAL MUSCLES—the muscles in the back of the neck—work together to turn the neck and to extend the head and neck, allowing you to look up and back. These two muscles need to be examined together because of their close working relationship. Both muscles run vertically in the back of the neck. Semispinalis capitis attaches to the base of the skull; it acts to extend the head. Semispinalis cervicis attaches to the neck and its primary action is on the neck. Semispinalis cervicis is one of the most powerful muscles of the neck; for this reason it is sometimes called the "workhorse muscle."

When trigger points are present in semispinalis capitis pain encircles the head, with its greatest intensity experienced at the temple and forehead over the eye. Think of a painful vice-like grip around your head that is focused over your eye. Semispinalis cervicis trigger points produce pain and soreness at the base of the skull and into the neck. When trigger points are present there will be difficulty dropping your head downward (flexing the head and neck) and looking up and back (extending the neck and head). You won't be able to do either comfortably.

The posterior cervicals are deep, lying beneath several layers of muscle, but when there are areas of tightness and constriction they can be felt through the upper layers of muscle. Lie on your back with your head supported by a pillow that is thick enough to prevent your head from being forced forward or dropped back. Place your fingers at the base of the skull on either side of the spine. Move your fingers from the base of the skull to the upper back, within the muscle mass just beside the spine. Feel for thick bands of muscle. These will be the tight bands within the posterior cervicals. You might feel particular areas of thickness about 1 to 2 inches below the base of the skull and then again 1 to 2 inches below that. Once you find those areas, just hold your pressure gently into the muscle. Relax your head and neck and breathe slowly. With patience you'll begin to feel the softening of the bands and the release of the muscle.

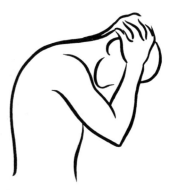

Stretch: Posterior cervicals

To stretch the posterior cervicals drop your head forward, aiming your chin for your chest. Allow the weight of your head to stretch these muscles. Hold this position for a count of ten to twenty. Repeat the stretch regularly throughout the day for a complete release.

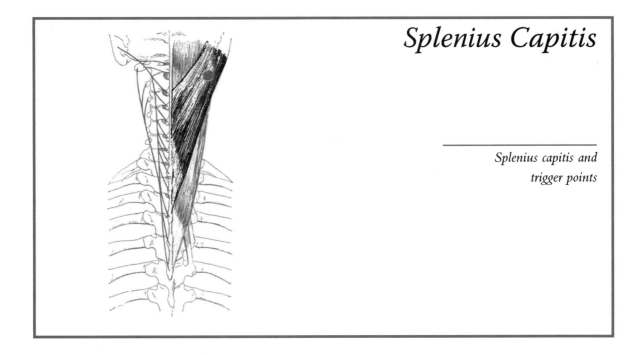

Splenius Capitis

Splenius capitis and trigger points

SPLENIUS CAPITIS lies beneath the trapezius. It runs diagonally from the base of the skull, at the bump that can be felt behind the ear, to the vertebrae in the middle of the neck and the upper back. The muscle may be difficult to feel. Splenius capitis extends the head and neck and turns it to the side.

Thrusting the head forward is the action that most often is the precursor of trigger points. Tennis players anticipating the serve have their heads in that position. When there are trigger points in splenius capitis the pain will be felt directly at the top of the head.

To locate and treat splenius capitis, sit with your back resting

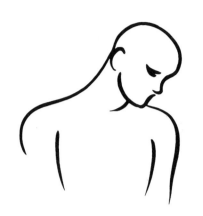

Stretch: Splenius capitis

against a chair. You'll want to find the space between the upper trapezius (page 42) and the sternocleidomastoid (page 28). First, locate the bump at the base of your skull behind the ear. The sternocleidomastoid starts there. Press just behind the SCM and move your hand down the side of the neck. You'll begin to feel the front border of the trapezius as you reach the middle of your neck. Just at that level, start to feel for a thin band of muscle in between the trapezius and the SCM. Gently press into that band. Hold it for several seconds to allow it to release. Work the trigger point in this way several times during the day. Follow it up with stretches.

To stretch splenius capitis, drop your head forward and down, turning the neck 20 to 30 degrees away from the painful side. Hold this position for a count of ten to twenty.

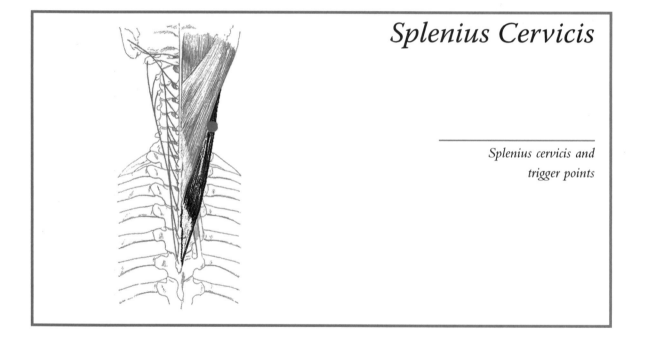

Splenius Cervicis

Splenius cervicis and trigger points

SPLENIUS CERVICIS attaches to the vertebrae of the neck and upper back. It extends the neck, turns the neck, and bends it to the side.

Thrusting the head forward is the action that most often is the source of trigger point development in this muscle: a tennis player anticipating receiving the serve has his or her head in this exact position. When there are trigger points in this muscle you may experience neck, head, and eye pain. Neck pain will be felt right at the angle of the neck, where the neck meets the shoulder, and it might include neck stiffness as well. There may even be some aching pain that goes through the head to the back of the eye. You might experience blurry vision in that eye as well.

Try to feel for splenius cervicis right at the angle of the neck. Sit with your back resting against a chair and bend your head, just a bit, to the side that the pain is on. You'll be able to slide your fingers in between two layers of muscle to touch the deeper splenius. Once you're able to feel the muscle, bend your head just a bit to the other side; you'll feel splenius tightening under your fingers. Press gently into that band, holding it for several seconds. You'll start to feel the muscle release slowly.

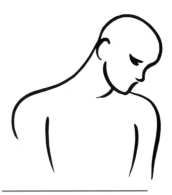

Stretch: Splenius cervicis

To stretch splenius cervicis, drop your head forward and down, turning the neck 30 to 40 degrees away from the painful side. Hold this position for a count of ten to twenty.

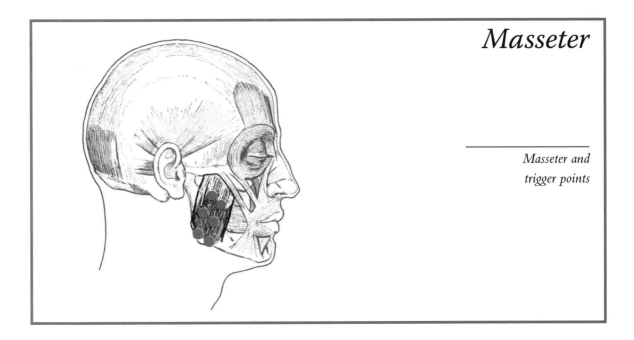

Masseter

Masseter and trigger points

THE MASSETER is one of the strongest muscles of the face. It attaches to the part of the cheekbone that is close to the ear and to the jawbone, the mandible. It works when you chew and clench your teeth by raising the lower jaw. If you place your hand on your cheek, just by your lower jaw, and gently clench your teeth, you will feel the masseter move as it contracts. You may be able to see it contracting and releasing when a person is angry and automatically clenches and releases his or her jaw.

If you consider the action of this muscle you can figure out what

Head and Face Pain

■

causes its restriction—clenching on a mouth guard; clenching on a regulator or snorkel; clenching the teeth at night. Periods of any such activity can easily trigger the restriction of the masseter. Bodybuilders naturally clench their teeth when they are lifting heavy weights. Everyday actions—biting on something hard, chewing gum, biting the nails—or sustaining a trauma to the head that involves the jaw can also cause trigger points to develop in the masseter.

When the masseter develops taut bands and trigger points, it can become the source of facial pain. Sometimes the pain will be felt over the upper teeth and cheek and above the eyebrow. Trigger point pain might be described as sinus pain and it may even be misdiagnosed as a sinus infection. Sometimes the pain will be felt on the side of your cheek and deep in the ear, and it may cause ringing in the ears. When the masseter develops trigger points you may not be able to open your mouth as wide as you would like. Normally you can open your mouth comfortably to accommodate the knuckles of two stacked fingers. If you can't do that, you have restriction in your jaw and you need to feel for trigger points in the masseter as well as in the other muscles involved in chewing: the temporalis and the pterygoids.

The masseter is covered by the parotid gland (the gland that swells when you get the mumps), so trigger points can sometimes be difficult to identify from the outside. You need to examine and treat the muscle from the inside of your cheek. Wash your hands well, then place your thumb on the inside of your mouth and your fingers on your cheek. Clench your teeth just a bit to identify the muscle. Use your thumb to work out any taut bands and sore spots in the muscle. It might be quite sore and painful; you may need to treat the muscle in this way several times during a day and over a period of days. Keep at it and it will release slowly. A good time to work on this muscle is when you're in the shower. Your muscle will be warmed up and your hands will be clean.

After you've worked on the muscle you need to stretch it out. Place your hand under your chin to provide mild resistance to opening your mouth. Open your mouth gently against that resistance. Hold the position for a count of three to five. Repeat this stretch three times. Following this stretch cycle, open and close your mouth several times without resistance.

It's important to avoid those activities that produce restriction in the jaw muscles—chewing gum, biting into hard foods, biting your nails, or clenching into a mouthpiece. Correcting a head-forward position is an important part of treating and retraining these muscles. Being mindful of the need to change is the first step toward lasting change.

You can begin to alter your head posture by trying to lengthen your spine, as if you were suspended from a string attached right at the top of your head. When seated you can place a small pillow or support at the small of your back in order to raise your chest. This will also allow your head to take on a more upright position.

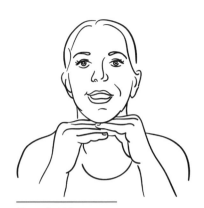

Stretch: Masseter

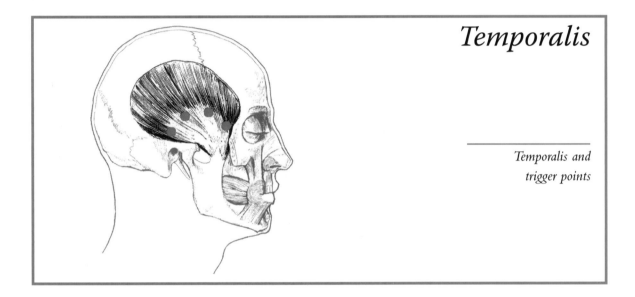

Temporalis

Temporalis and trigger points

THE TEMPORALIS is the strongest and most efficient of the chewing muscles. Temporalis is a large, flat muscle that lies on the temple, fanning the ear. Its lower attachment is to the jawbone, the mandible. Temporalis works with the masseter to close the jaw. If you place your fingers above your ears on your temples and lightly clench your back teeth you will be able to feel the contraction of temporalis.

Trigger points can develop in the temporalis much in the same way that they develop in the masseter—through clenching the teeth, grinding the teeth, and direct trauma caused by an impact or a fall. When trigger points do develop, pain is experienced as a headache in the temple region and it may extend as far as the eyebrow, the upper teeth, and to the area of the temporomandibular joint (TMJ). In addition to pain, your teeth might feel hypersensitive to heat, cold, or pressure. If your teeth are painful it's important to see a dentist, but if the dentist

Head and Face Pain

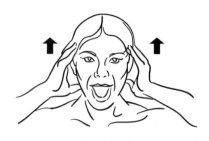

Stretch: Temporalis

is unable to identify anything wrong with the tooth it's clearly worth your time and effort to try to find and release taut bands and trigger points in the temporalis muscle.

You can locate temporalis trigger points by spreading your fingertips in an arc about one inch above your ear and into the temple. Lightly clench your back teeth. You will feel the muscular contraction under your fingers. Gently move your fingers back and forth across the fibers of the muscle to locate taut bands within it. The trigger points will be the most sensitive points within those taut bands. Compress the points gently for several seconds to release them.

To stretch temporalis spread your fingers across the muscle, just behind the temples and above the ears. Open your mouth as wide as you can and inhale; as you exhale, press upward along the course of the fibers of the muscle. Hold for a count of five to ten. Repeat several times.

Just as with masseter, it's important to avoid those actions that produce restriction in the muscles involved with chewing—chewing gum, biting into hard foods, biting your nails, or clenching a mouthpiece.

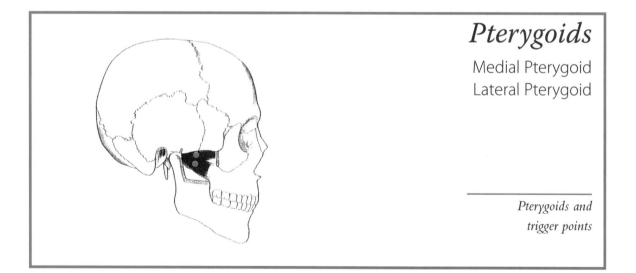

Pterygoids
Medial Pterygoid
Lateral Pterygoid

*Pterygoids and
trigger points*

THE PTERYGOIDS suspend the lower jaw from their bony attachments within the skull. They work with the masseter and the temporalis to elevate the jaw, they produce the back-and-forth motion needed to grind food, and they draw the jawbone forward, a movement that's necessary for opening the jaw wide.

The lateral pterygoid is the most common muscular source of TMJ dysfunction, yet the pterygoids are often overlooked because of the nature of the symptoms that are associated with trigger point development. Pain in the cheekbone and temporomandibular joint just in front of the ear, painful clicking of the jaw when opening and closing the mouth, difficulty in opening the mouth wide, and chewing difficulties send people to dentists and TMJ specialists, not myofascial therapists. Sinus pain with increased mucus production from the sinuses send patients to an ear, nose and throat doctor. In fact, all of these symptoms are associated with a muscular source of restriction.

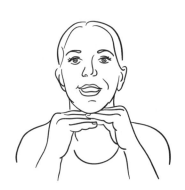

Stretch: Lateral pterygoid

The pterygoids are small muscles and their position is well back on the jaw, so they are difficult to feel. To find the lateral pterygoid, start at the cheekbone just in front of the ear. Press the underside of the cheekbone, following its course toward your nose. Open and close your jaw as you do this and you'll feel the lateral pterygoid contract and release about an inch away from your ear. If there are trigger points you will feel a very tender, tight vertical band reaching up underneath your cheekbone. Press right into that band.

You can work on the lower end of the medial pterygoid by pressing up underneath the angle of the jaw about $1/2$ inch. The upper fibers of medial pterygoid need to be reached inside your mouth. Wash your hands and then reach way into the back of your mouth, behind your last molar. You'll feel the sharp, bony edge of the jawbone. Work on the muscle just behind that. Gently biting down on a small object such as a pencil or a cork will help you to identify the muscle clearly. If there are restrictions in the muscle it will undoubtedly be very sore. Work for brief periods of time several times throughout the day.

Follow up with a stretch. Place your hand under your chin to provide a mild resistance to opening your mouth. Open your mouth gently against that resistance. Hold the position for a count of three to five. Repeat this three times. Following this stretch cycle, open and close your mouth several times without resistance.

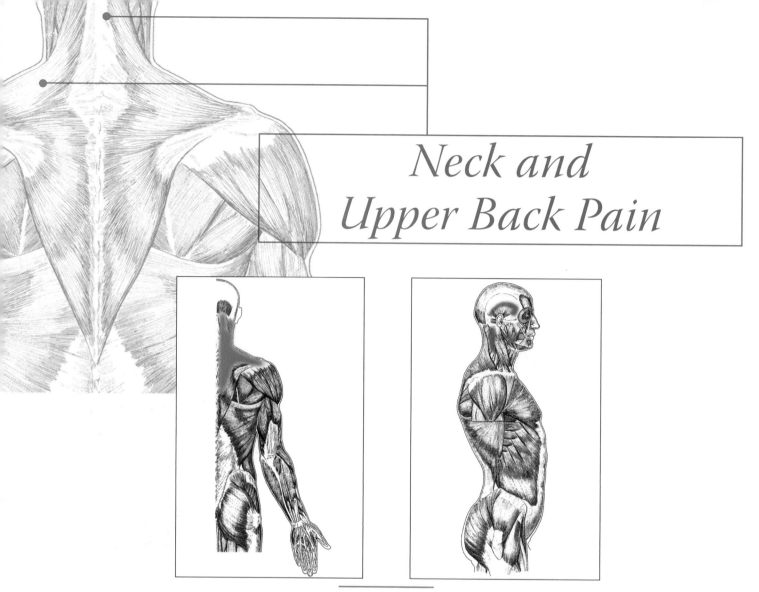

Neck and Upper Back Pain

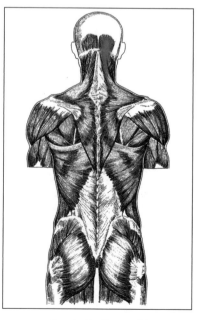

Pain pattern: Trapezius

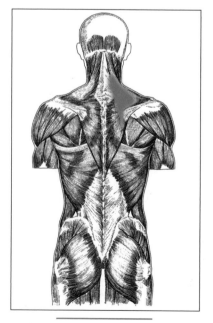

Pain pattern: Levator scapulae

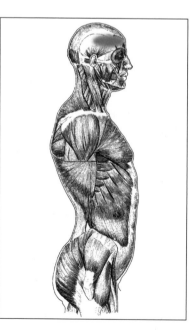

Semispinalis capitis

Semispinalis cervicis

Pain pattern: Posterior cervicals

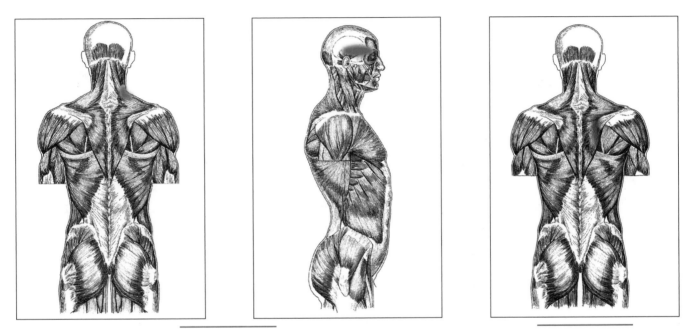

Pain pattern: Splenius cervicis

Pain pattern: Rhomboids

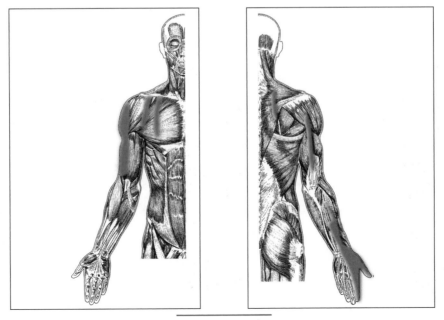

Pain pattern: Scalenes

The human body is an astounding structure, and the neck is a mighty example of that truth. Stacked upon the spinal column of the torso lie the seven vertebrae that form the bony structure of the neck and serve to support the head. There are numerous muscles that act on the neck and head that provide its means of movement. Some are a continuation of muscles that are placed on the back; some are specific to the neck itself. The complex design of muscle and bone makes the neck capable of intricate movements and gives it the strength to support the approximately eight-pound weight of the human head. For all of its intricacy, though—or perhaps because of it—the neck is subject to muscular stresses that often lead to pain and dysfunction.

The sources of trigger point development in the musculature of the neck are quite numerous: overload, overwork, trauma, compromising postures, and emotional stresses are just some of them. Overload may occur from the many activities that strain the neck muscles. Keeping the head and neck in the same position for a sustained period of time can lead to restriction and associated trigger points. This might occur when you're painting a ceiling or sitting in the front rows at the movies or the theater. Working at a computer station at which your monitor is off to one side can encourage trigger point development for the prolonged neck rotation that such a set-up demands. Sleeping on several pillows or a pillow that is either too thick or too flat can lead to restriction in the muscles; falling asleep while lying on your side with your head on the arm of a couch is a classic position that overloads the neck muscles, leading to pain and stiffness and limiting range of motion in the neck.

Many dancers and athletes "stretch" their necks improperly, over-stretching or straining the muscles in the process. Neck rolls, for example, place undue stress on the smaller muscles of the neck, requiring these muscles to support the weight of the head at certain points during the roll, which causes them to become overloaded. Trigger points may result as a function of this overload.

Equally problematic is the head-forward posture: chin jutting out, the muscles in the back of the neck shortening. This is a common posture for bicyclists when they're riding; it's a familiar posture for football players and tennis players as well. A round-shouldered upper-body posture, common in weight lifters with overdeveloped chest muscles, large-breasted women, and elderly people of both genders, may also result in a head-forward position; this easily leads to overload injury to the neck muscles.

Whiplash-type injuries, the sudden forward and then backward motion of the neck experienced during a tackle or fall or a sideways impact, are common sources of neck injury. Football players, or any athlete who is at risk of a fall or impact, might experience trauma to the muscles of the neck.

Another common source of neck injury is improper breathing. Breathing high into the chest rather than into the lower belly causes the muscles of the neck to become involved in breathing, leading to a state of chronic overuse. Stress, of course, does the same thing—a great deal of tension can become locked in the neck, throat, upper chest, and shoulders. Stress alone is a primary source of trigger point development in muscles affecting the neck and upper back.

If you are suffering with neck pain, consider the sources of your pain. Is the pain a result of your physical activities? your posture? the life stresses you embody? an inefficient breathing pattern? The pain may come from more than one source. You will have to address them all in order to find true resolution and make your neck pain free.

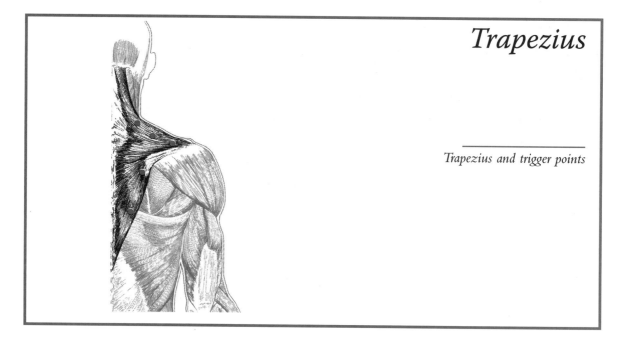

Trapezius

Trapezius and trigger points

OF ALL THE MUSCLES in the body, trapezius is the one that most frequently develops trigger points. Trapezius attaches to the base of the skull and lies at the back of the neck, the upper shoulders, and over the upper and middle back. Trapezius is actually comprised of three different groups of fibers: an upper group, a middle group, and a lower group. The muscle fibers of upper trapezius drape across the upper shoulders to attach to the collarbone (the clavicle) on the upper chest. The upper trapezius forms the characteristic shape of the upper shoulder area that is closest to the neck. This muscle is the only muscle in the body that raises the tip of the shoulders, producing the "shrug." The upper trapezius also moves the head and neck toward the shoulder on the same side.

The fibers of the middle trapezius pull the shoulder blades together. The fibers of the lower trapezius draw the shoulder blades downward.

Trigger points can develop in many different areas of the trapezius, causing pain in various places in the neck and upper back. Trigger points commonly develop as a result of overload, compression, and trauma. Stress is often the greatest source of overload. If you think about your posture when you're stressed you will see that your shoulders often bear the biggest burden; you seem to wear your shoulders around your ears. It is this shoulders-to-the-ears posture that trapezius is responsible for. It's not for nothing that we speak of carrying the weight of the world on our shoulders—when we do "carry the world" this way, it's the trapezius that is affected. Overload also occurs as a function of continually raising your shoulder to your ear, as you might do to hold a phone between the two.

Trapezius is the muscle that supports the weight of your arms. When you are seated on a chair without arm support, the trapezius works continually to support your arm weight. The dancer practicing overhead lifts, the weight lifter doing military presses, and the cyclist bent over her handlebars are all in danger of developing trapezius trigger points due to overload of the muscle.

Compressing the trapezius also leads to trigger points: hikers whose backpacks are ill fitted or those who carry heavy gear on their shoulders may risk developing trigger points from compression. Trauma in the form of whiplash—the forceful, unexpected, and uncontrolled forward-then-backward motion of the head—frequently produces trigger points. Auto accidents are a well-known cause of whiplash injuries. So are falls, something that any one of us may experience.

Pain from trigger points in the upper trapezius is felt on the side of the neck up to the base of the skull, possibly traveling around the ear to the temple. The pain is often described as deep and achy. You may experience this pain pattern as a headache, particularly when pain is felt in the temples. Trigger points in the middle fibers of trapezius don't occur frequently, but when they do they refer pain between the shoulder blades close to the spine. Trigger points in the lower fibers refer pain to the back of the neck.

Trigger points occur far more frequently in upper trapezius than in either the middle or lower fibers. To find trigger points in the upper trapezius, sit on a chair with your elbow supported. The trapezius supports the weight of the entire arm, so you want your arm to be supported by the arm of the chair to get the weight off the trapezius and to allow it to relax. Feel the top of your shoulder, between the outside edge of the shoulder and your ear. You can grasp the muscle between your fingers and thumb—it's thick. There will be trigger points in the front of the muscle as well as the back of the muscle, so first seek out bands and soreness in the front of the muscle before you move on to working on the back of the muscle. When trigger points are present you will feel bands of muscle that hurt; you may even feel individual "knots" that, when pressed, refer pain right up the side of your neck to the base of the skull. When you find one of these points, use your fingers to press in to the point where you feel

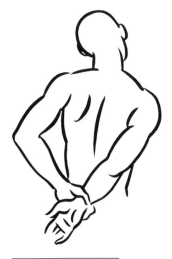

Stretch 1: Trapezius

Neck and
Upper Back Pain

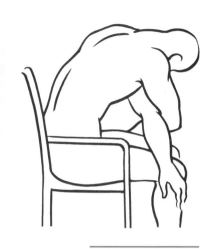

Stretch 2: Trapezius

tenderness and pain. Breathe and relax your chest and arms. After several seconds pass you'll begin to feel the muscle softening and the knots release. Repeat this treatment several times over the course of the day. The more frequently you work on the muscle the more it will release, and it will hold the release longer and longer.

To release trigger points in the middle and lower fibers of trapezius, lie on the floor and place a tennis ball or a ball of similar size on the area of the muscle where you feel the most soreness. Allow the weight of your body to compress the ball against your back. Breathe and relax and let gravity and the ball do the job of releasing the trigger point.

Stretch upper trapezius after working on it to gain the greatest relief. Bend your head away from the painful side, aiming your ear for your shoulder. Hold this position for a count of ten to twenty. To increase the stretch, grasp the wrist of the arm on the painful side behind your back and gently pull it toward the painless side.

To stretch middle and lower trapezius, sit in a chair. Bend forward with your head dropped. Cross each arm over the body to grasp the opposite knee. Hold this position for a count of ten to twenty.

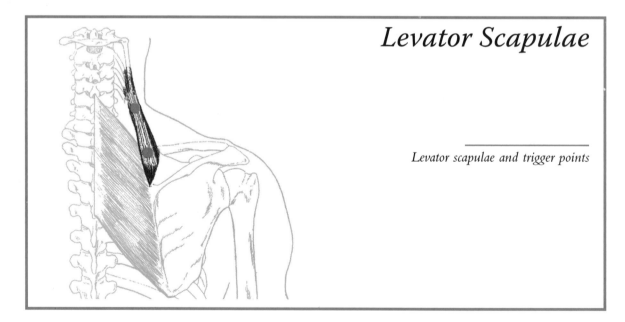

Levator Scapulae

Levator scapulae and trigger points

LEVATOR SCAPULAE is one of the most commonly involved muscles, second only to the trapezius in being both a source of neck pain and a frequent location at which trigger points develop. Levator scapulae lies underneath the trapezius. It attaches to the upper vertebrae of the neck and to the inner corner of the shoulder blade. As its name describes, when the levator scapulae contracts it elevates the scapula (in lay terms, it raises the shoulder blade). It also works with other muscles to rotate and bend the neck.

A common cause of trigger points in levator scapulae is keeping your head in one position for an extended period of time: holding the phone between your ear and your shoulder, working on a computer or watching television where the screen is off to one side, and falling asleep on your side with pillows that are too high are all examples of positions that can cause trigger points to develop if the position is held for too long. The stresses of hiking your shoulders up and holding your head in a forward posture affect levator scapulae—whether these muscular stresses are generated during sport or are simply postural habits, they are nonetheless recipes for levator scapulae trigger points. If you watch your posture when you are emotionally stressed you will see that your shoulders somehow manage to hike themselves up close to your ears; this is another common source of trigger points in levator scapulae.

When trigger points are present in the levator scapulae, pain will be felt at the angle of the neck where the neck and the shoulder meet. There might also be some pain in the upper back, just between the shoulder blade and the spine. The hallmark of active levator scapulae trigger points is a stiff neck that won't let you turn your head fully to the same side as the pain. If this is one of your symptoms, work on levator scapulae first!

To feel taut bands and trigger points in levator scapulae, you'll have to feel through the trapezius. Use the hand on the side opposite the pain to reach over your painful shoulder. Lift that shoulder up and drop it down and you'll feel the movement of your shoulder blade. Once you feel the inside edge of the shoulder blade, move your hand a bit closer to the spine. If there are trigger points in levator scapulae, you will feel a ropelike band of muscle that has a sore spot that both hurts and feels good when you press it. Stretch your neck over to the opposite side as you do this. At first you might feel a burning sensation—if you do you'll know that you're in the right place. Work on the trigger points in the muscle and you will feel it slowly release.

To stretch levator scapulae, bend your head away from the painful side, aiming your ear toward your shoulder. Rotate your face approximately 30 degrees away from the painful side and then drop

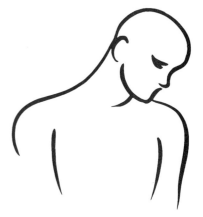

Stretch: Levator scapulae

your head down slightly, aiming your chin for your chest. Hold this position for a count of ten to twenty.

Once this muscle is released, watch what you do. Figure out whether it's activity, posture, or stress that aggravates the muscle, and then try to correct the situation to avoid developing trigger points in levator scapulae in the future.

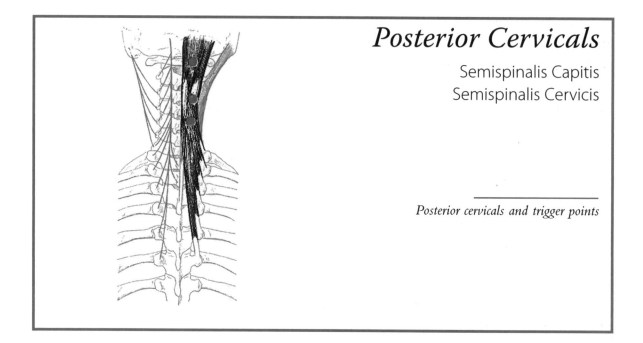

Posterior Cervicals

Semispinalis Capitis
Semispinalis Cervicis

Posterior cervicals and trigger points

THE POSTERIOR CERVICAL MUSCLES—the muscles in the back of the neck—work together to turn the neck and to extend the head and neck, allowing you to look up and back. These two muscles need to be examined together because of their close working relationship. Both muscles run vertically in the back of the neck. Semispinalis capitis attaches to the base of the skull; it acts to extend the head. Semispinalis cervicis attaches to the neck and its primary action is on the neck. Semispinalis cervicis is one of the most powerful muscles of the neck; for this reason it is sometimes called the "workhorse muscle."

When trigger points are present in semispinalis capitis, pain encircles the head, with its greatest intensity experienced at the temple and forehead over the eye. Think of a painful vice-like grip around your head that is focused over your eye. Semispinalis cervicis trigger points produce pain and soreness at the base of the skull and into the neck. When trigger points are present there will be difficulty dropping your head downward (flexing the head and neck) and looking up and back (extending the neck and head). You won't be able to do either comfortably.

The posterior cervicals are deep, lying beneath several layers of muscle, but when there are areas of tightness and constriction they can be felt through the upper layers of muscle. Lie on your back with your head supported by a pillow that is thick enough to prevent your head from being forced forward or dropped back. Place your fingers at the base of the skull on either side of the spine. Move your fingers from the base of the skull to the upper back, within the muscle mass just beside the spine. Feel for thick bands of muscle. These will be the tight bands within the posterior cervicals. You might feel particular areas of thickness about 1 to 2 inches below the base of the skull and then again 1 to 2 inches below that. Once you find those areas, just hold your pressure gently into the muscle. Relax your head and neck and breathe slowly. With patience you'll begin to feel the softening of the bands and the release of the muscle.

To stretch the posterior cervicals drop your head forward, aiming your chin for your chest. Allow the weight of your head to stretch these muscles. Hold this position for a count of ten to twenty. Repeat the stretch regularly throughout the day for a complete release.

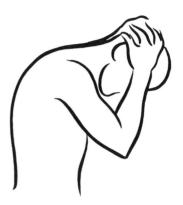

Stretch: Posterior cervicals

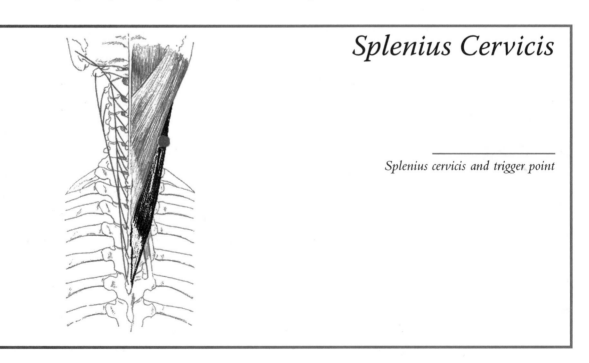

Splenius Cervicis

Splenius cervicis and trigger point

SPLENIUS CERVICIS attaches to the vertebrae of the neck and upper back. It extends the neck, turns the neck, and bends it to the side.

Thrusting the head forward is the action that most often is the

Neck and
Upper Back Pain

■

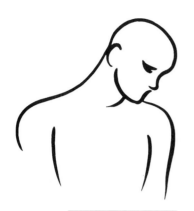

Stretch: Splenius cervicis

source of trigger point development in this muscle: a tennis player anticipating receiving the serve has his head in this exact position. When there are trigger points in this muscle you may experience neck, head, and eye pain. Neck pain will be felt right at the angle of the neck, where the neck meets the shoulder, and it might include neck stiffness as well. There may even be some aching pain that goes through the head to the back of the eye. You might experience blurry vision in that eye as well.

Try to feel for splenius cervicis right at the angle of the neck. Sit with your back resting against a chair and bend your head, just a bit, to the side that the pain is on. You'll be able to slide your fingers in between two layers of muscle to touch the deeper splenius. Once you're able to feel the muscle, bend your head just a bit to the other side; you'll feel splenius tightening under your fingers. Press gently into that band, holding it for several seconds. You'll start to feel the muscle release slowly.

To stretch splenius cervicis, drop your head forward and down, turning the neck 30 to 40 degrees away from the painful side. Hold this position for a count of ten to twenty.

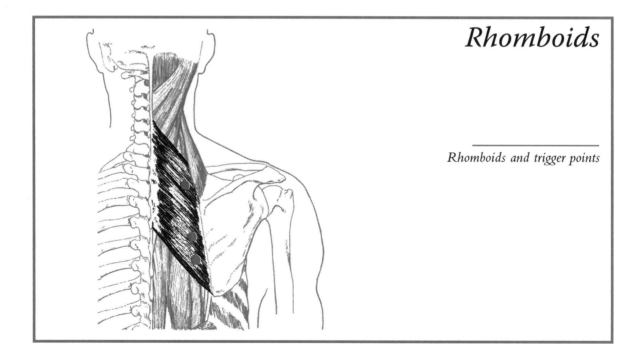

Rhomboids

Rhomboids and trigger points

LYING JUST BENEATH the trapezius, the rhomboids connect the shoulder blades to the vertebrae of the upper back. In concert with the middle fibers of trapezius, the rhomboids draw the shoulder blades together. They also elevate the shoulder blades, along with levator scapulae.

The rhomboids tend toward weakness, particularly when the pectoralis major on the front of the chest is overworked or very tight. Pectoralis major is the muscle in the upper chest that gives that part of the body its shapely look; see page 62. Many weight lifters and bodybuilders overwork the pectoral muscles and as a result they end up with a round-shouldered look: the force of the overworked pectorals draws the shoulders forward and the consequent pull on the rhomboids causes the rhomboids to weaken and develop trigger points. Any kind of work that has you leaning forward in a round-shoulder position will put the rhomboids at risk for trigger points.

Pain coming from trigger points in the rhomboids is a superficial ache felt along the inner border of the shoulder blades. The pain is completely unaffected by movement; you will feel it whether you are resting or moving. A pain pattern involving the rhomboids is never about the rhomboids alone. You will only recognize that the rhomboids are involved once you've eliminated trigger points in trapezius, levator scapulae, and infraspinatus. If you hear or feel a snapping or crunching noise when you move your shoulder blades, the rhomboids are involved. Upper back pain can be due to rhomboid trigger points as well.

The easiest way to release trigger points in the rhomboids is to lie on the floor with a ball placed on the muscle between the shoulder blade and the spine. You may need to support your head on a thin pillow for comfort. You'll know exactly where the ball needs to be when you lie on it and experience the soreness of a compressed trigger point. As you lie on the floor let your body relax. Breathe deep and let gravity do the work.

Stretch the rhomboids after you've worked on them. Sit in a chair and bend forward with your head dropped. Cross each arm over your body to grasp the opposite knee. Hold this position for a count of ten to twenty.

To help counteract a round-shouldered position when you're sitting you might use a lumbar support at your low back, just above your waist, to help raise your upper chest and drop your shoulder blades. A rolled towel works well for this purpose too.

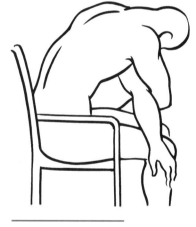

Stretch: Rhomboids

Neck and
Upper Back Pain

49

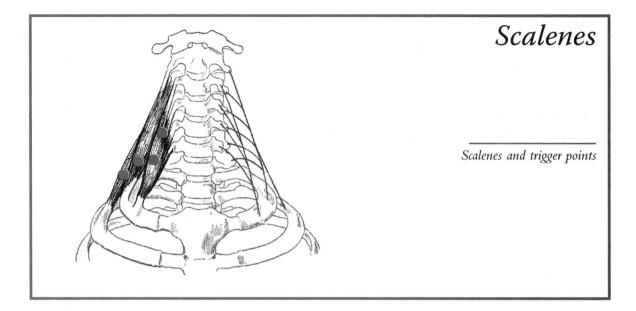

Scalenes and trigger points

THE SCALENES are comprised of three small muscles on the side of the neck that work to bend the neck to the side and to stabilize the neck against sideways impact. Because they attach to the first and second ribs, they are also active in raising the upper rib cage to assist in breathing.

Scalene trigger points are a frequent source of shoulder and arm pain. These small muscles help to support and raise the upper rib cage when carrying, lifting, or pulling heavy objects, particularly with the arms at the level of the waist. Straining to do any of these activities is a source of trigger points. So is carrying the weight of a heavy backpack on the shoulders instead of the hips.

Any force that can produce a whiplash is a source of injury to the scalenes, whether that force is from an automobile accident, a fall, or an impact in contact sports. Breathing high into your chest or holding your breath up in the chest strongly activates the scalenes and can lead to the development of trigger points. We're all guilty of breathing like this, particularly when we're learning a new skill or when we're working hard or feeling highly stressed. Suffering with either chronic or acute breathing problems such as emphysema, pneumonia, bronchitis, or chronic cough can also contribute to the development of trigger points in the scalenes.

Trigger points in the scalenes produce a complex pain pattern that is deep, aching, and persistent. Pain can be experienced in the upper chest and/or the upper back; it can be experienced in the side or back of the shoulder and arm and on the thumb side of the arm and hand, including the thumb and index finger. The pain can be in all of these places or it can be in only one of them, and the location of pain can change from one day to the next. In addition to pain you might feel weakness in the hand and arm that makes you drop things unexpectedly.

The scalenes are often overlooked as the source of these various pain patterns. You can test yourself to see if the scalenes are responsible for your pain. Turn your head fully to the side of your pain and then drop your chin in toward your collarbone. If your pain increases it's a sign that trigger points in the scalenes are the cause.

The scalenes are hard to visualize and difficult to feel. Look in the mirror. Tilt your head to the right. As the scalenes contract you'll be able to see the right sternocleidomastoid muscle spanning from underneath your ear to your collarbone. Using your left hand, place the tips of three fingers just behind the sternocleidomastoid at about its midpoint (see page 28) and then straighten your head, keeping your neck relaxed. Press very, very gently back and forth just behind the SCM and you may feel the very thin, taut bands of the scalenes. Once you've found the taut bands try to isolate them under your fingertips, then press very slowly and gently. There are many delicate structures in the front of the neck: you must approach this area with a cautious touch. Even so, once you've found the scalenes you will be able to release them.

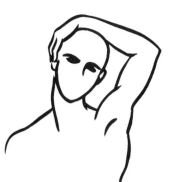
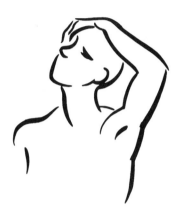
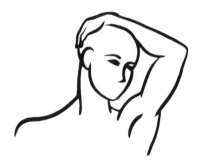

Stretch: Scalenes

Once you've worked on the scalenes, stretching them is essential. Bend your head and neck, aiming the ear of your painless side toward that same shoulder. Hold this position for a count of ten. Then, without changing the angle of your head, rotate your head and face toward the painful side, stretching your cheek toward the ceiling. Hold this position for a count of ten. Return your head and face to the initial position. Now rotate the head and face again, this time aiming your chin for your collarbone. Hold this position for a count of ten before returning it to the initial position. Slowly release your neck from the stretch. You may feel that you are a bit stiffer stretching up rather than stretching down, or vice versa. This tells you which direction needs the most stretch. Remember: these are delicate areas and the stretch, like the touch, has to be gentle. Nonetheless, your work will be effective if you keep at it.

Once you've released the trigger points in the scalenes, work on retraining your breath, breathing deeply into your lower abdomen rather than up into your chest. See page 173 for the specifics on how to do this.

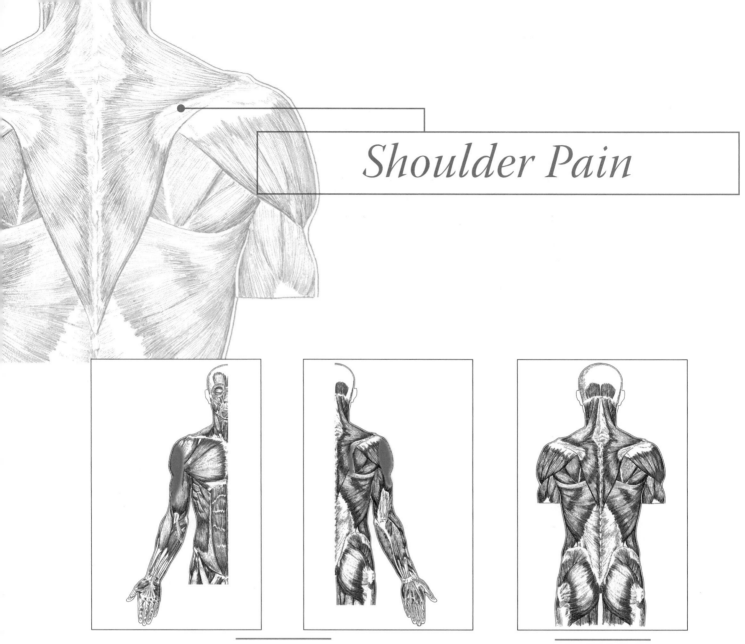

Shoulder Pain

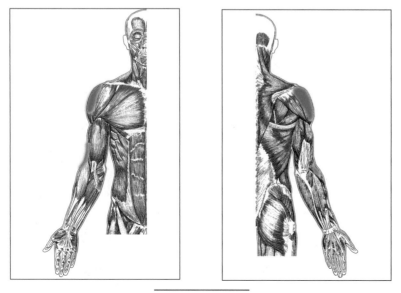

Pain pattern: Infraspinatus

Pain pattern: Teres minor

Pain pattern: Supraspinatus

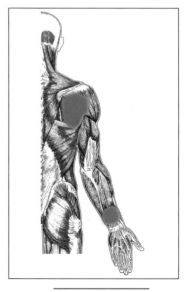

Pain pattern: Subscapularis

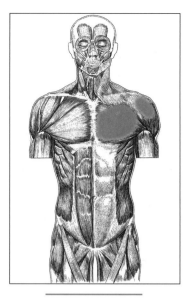

Pain pattern: Pectoralis major

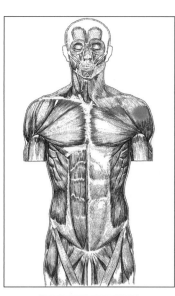

Pain pattern: Pectoralis minor

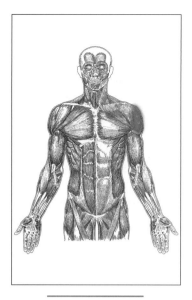

Pain pattern: Deltoid

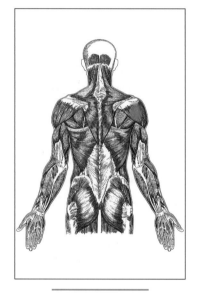

Pain pattern: Deltoid

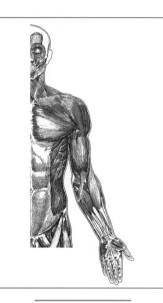

Pain pattern: Biceps brachii

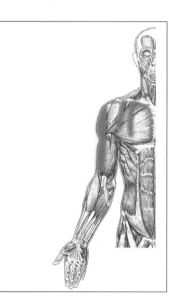

Pain pattern: Scalenes

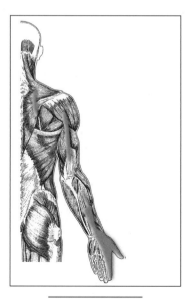

Pain pattern: Scalenes

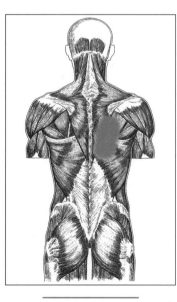

Pain pattern: Latissimus dorsi

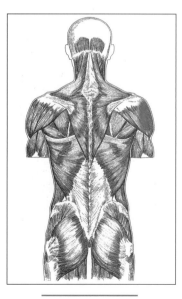

Pain pattern: Teres major

If you place your hand on the area where the humerus, the long bone of the upper arm, meets your torso, you will be touching your shoulder joint. If you move your arm around you will be able to feel the motion of the head of the humerus at the joint. But the shoulder region encompasses a much larger area. Considering the shoulder as a whole requires looking at the muscles of the upper chest and upper back and the muscles that form the axilla, the armpit. In other words, the shoulder cannot be separated from the torso. Portions of the clavicle (collarbone), the scapula (shoulder blade), and humerus form the bony components of the shoulder joint. More than a dozen muscles provide its action. The extraordinary construction of the shoulder joint allows for its extensive range of motion, atypical of any other joint in the body. Yet it is this very construction that makes the shoulder joint one of the most unstable and easily injured areas in the body.

Injuries to the shoulder occur to both athletes and nonathletes alike, and the sources of these injuries are numerous. Muscular strain can occur from the simplest action, something as seemingly inconsequential as reaching back to grasp the seat belt in your car or turning off the light switch beside your bed. Preventing an unexpected fall by reaching out and landing on your arm is frequently the source of shoulder injury, and pulling against the leash while walking a large dog or carrying a heavy bag at your side can strain the muscles of your shoulder as well. And think about the frequent air traveler. He or she often uses invariably heavy carry-on luggage that must be pulled from behind through long airport walkways. Once travelers are on board the airplane they must lift the carry-on bag, often awkwardly and in a confined space, to place it in an overhead compartment. Once air travelers have reached their seats it is not unreasonable to suspect that some strain has occurred to the shoulder muscles.

Shoulder injury is only too common in sports and dance, and often the reason for injury is chronic overuse, sudden muscular strain, or practicing your sport using poor technique. Four of the muscles acting on the shoulder joint are those muscles that comprise the rotator cuff: supraspinatus, infraspinatus, teres minor, and subscapularis. They are directly involved in the rotation of the shoulder and upper arm. The muscles that provide the power for that movement are the deltoid muscle, which caps the shoulder joint; pectoralis major, which lies on the front of the chest; and latissimus dorsi, which passes from the low back and side of the torso before attaching onto the upper arm. These large and powerful muscles are easily injured through the overuse that so many athletes subject their bodies to during periods of intense training.

Shoulder injury is common in baseball and football—pitchers, outfielders, and quarterbacks are repeatedly throwing the ball as long and as far as they can, sometimes exhausting the muscles in practice. In tennis and volleyball it's the overhand serve that does the job on the shoulder; swimmers rotate their shoulders and arms in just about every stroke. Weight lifters and wrestlers will sometimes overload these muscles by lifting overhead something (or someone) that is heavier than the muscles are capable of carrying. Watch the male dancer as he lifts and carries his partner or catches her as she leaps across the floor into his arms. To provide the appearance of effortlessness he has practiced that lift hundreds of times, each time putting strain on his shoulders, arms, chest, and back; he is at risk for an overuse injury. Any athlete in any sport who is not practicing "clean" technique involving the shoulder and arm is at risk of straining these muscles.

Because of the interrelationship of the muscles working on this joint, when one muscle is injured all the muscles that act on the shoulder joint may be affected. These include pectoralis major, pectoralis minor, the rhomboids, and serratus anterior, as well as several muscles that act on the arm: biceps brachii, latissimus dorsi, and teres major. Therefore it is recommended that each muscle in this group be palpated for taut bands, tenderness, and trigger points.

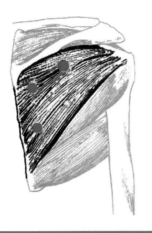

Infraspinatus

Infraspinatus and trigger points

THE ROTATOR CUFF is formed by the attachments of four muscles: infraspinatus, teres minor, supraspinatus, and subscapularis. Trigger points in these muscles are considered to be the most frequent source of shoulder pain and restricted motion in the shoulder joint. Each of the muscles attaches to the shoulder blade and to the head of the humerus at the upper arm. As a group they act on the upper arm to rotate it internally and externally and to maintain the position and stability of the shoulder joint when the arm is in motion.

Infraspinatus and teres minor externally rotate the upper arm, turning your palms outward. Infraspinatus lies on the shoulder blade (the scapula). The shoulder blade is a flat bone located on the upper part of your back and shoulder. Feel the flat, bony edge at the tip of your shoulder. That's the acromion, the outside edge of the shoulder blade. Follow that bone around to the back and you'll be on the part of the scapula called the spine of the scapula. It's just below this that the infraspinatus attaches.

If you trace the edge of the scapula outward to the shoulder and then externally rotate your arm a few times you'll be able to feel movement of the head of the humerus, the long bone of the upper arm. It's at the humerus that all the rotator cuff muscles attach. Infraspinatus covers the flat outer surface of the shoulder blade and then attaches to the upper arm at the head of the humerus. Trigger points in infraspinatus lie about one inch below the spine of the scapula, the most frequent trigger point being about an inch away from the inner edge of the shoulder blade itself.

Infraspinatus is the most frequent muscular source of shoulder pain. In fact, it is the third most frequently involved muscle in the body—only upper trapezius and levator scapulae develop trigger points more frequently. Because it is so often involved, it is here that you should start feeling for trigger points when your shoulder pain is either in the front or the back of your arm, covering the area where the deltoid is and slightly lower into the upper arm. The pain may feel very deep in the shoulder joint, and reaching behind your back could be very painful and difficult—you might be unable to reach into your back pocket or fasten a back button. You might not be able to sleep on either side when you have trigger points in this muscle; sleeping on the "good" side is as uncomfortable as sleeping on the "bad" side. Your arm might feel a bit weak; a tennis player with trigger points in the infraspinatus won't have any strength in the overhand serve.

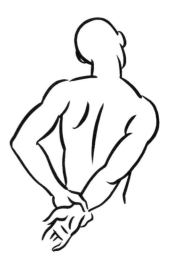

Stretch 1: Infraspinatus

The easiest way to release trigger points in infraspinatus is by using a small ball, such as a squash ball, instead of a finger to compress the muscle. Lie on your back on the floor. Place the ball between the upper part of your shoulder blade and the floor, positioning it at the place that you feel is the most sore when you press on it. That would be the trigger point. As you're lying down, just breathe and relax. It will take some time, maybe even several minutes, and it may require repeated attempts, but with patience the point will become less sensitive, indicating that the muscle is releasing.

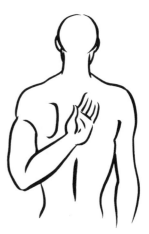

Stretch 2: Infraspinatus

Stretch infraspinatus and teres minor together. Reach behind your back at the level of the waist. Grasp the wrist of that arm with your other hand and gently pull the arm across your waist and then up slightly. Hold this position for a count of fifteen to twenty. As your flexibility increases, reach the fingers of that arm up toward the opposite shoulder blade. Another good stretch for these two muscles is to pull the arm across the chest. Hold it in this position for fifteen to twenty seconds, then release.

It's a good idea to work on each muscle of the rotator cuff if you have pain and restriction of shoulder movement that you suspect is caused by trigger points. Feel for restrictions and trigger points in each muscle and then take your arm through the range of stretches suggested for each muscle. Focusing on the group, rather than on one muscle within the group, is an effective means of regaining complete, pain-free use of your shoulder.

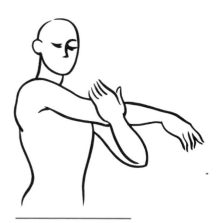

Stretch 3: Infraspinatus

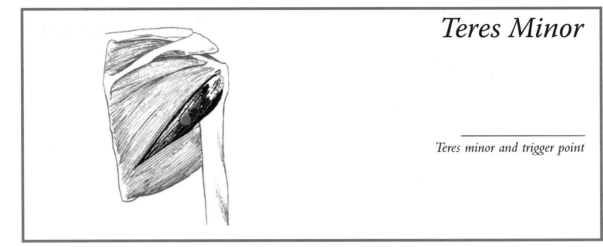

Teres Minor

Teres minor and trigger point

TERES MINOR is a small muscle that assists infraspinatus in externally rotating the arm. It lies just below infraspinatus, attaching to the shoulder blade on its outer edge and to the head of the humerus just below infraspinatus.

Unlike infraspinatus, teres minor does not develop trigger points very frequently, and when it does the pain is not associated with restricted motion in the arm. Pain is the back of the arm, just over the deltoid area; you usually notice it only after pain from trigger points in infraspinatus is relieved.

To find teres minor, reach under your arm to the back portion of your armpit. You will feel the sharp outside edge of the shoulder blade. Externally rotate your arm and you will feel the movement of teres minor as it contracts. Return your arm to a relaxed position and you will feel teres minor release. Press on the muscle; you will find a sore, tender point. Hold this point for several seconds to begin to feel the release of the muscle.

Stretch infraspinatus and teres minor together. Reach behind your back at the level of the waist. Grasp the wrist of that arm with your other hand and gently pull the arm across your waist and then up slightly. Hold this position for a count of fifteen to twenty. As your flexibility increases, reach the fingers of the affected arm up toward the opposite shoulder blade. Another good stretch for these two muscles is to pull the affected arm across the chest. Hold it in this position for fifteen to twenty seconds and release.

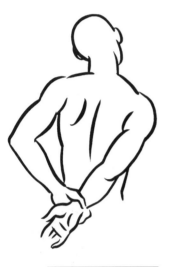

Stretch 1: Teres minor

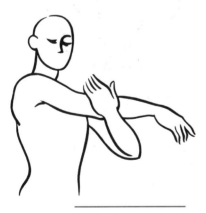

Stretch 2: Teres minor

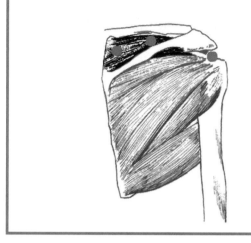

Supraspinatus

Supraspinatus and trigger points

SUPRASPINATUS is a small, thick muscle that lies in the horizontal depression in the upper part of the shoulder blade. Supraspinatus stabilizes the shoulder joint and works with the deltoid muscle to raise your arm to the side. Like the other rotator cuff muscles, it attaches to the upper part of the humerus. It lies deep underneath the fibers of the upper trapezius; because of its placement it might be a bit difficult to feel. Like infraspinatus, restrictions in supraspinatus are a common source of shoulder pain.

Trigger points develop in supraspinatus usually in combination with restriction in trapezius and infraspinatus. Carrying something quite heavy with your arms hanging at your side and pulling back against a forward tug are common instigators of trigger points. Rowers and weight lifters are at risk for trigger points at supraspinatus. Pain is usually in the area of the upper shoulder, right by the middle portion of the deltoid. The pain radiates down into the upper arm, sometimes to the forearm and the outside of the elbow. If there are trigger points in supraspinatus you may not be able to reach up to shave or comb your hair or reach back to place your hand into a back pocket or fasten a back button.

Trigger points in supraspinatus are a little difficult to locate because of muscle's location under trapezius. You will most likely need somebody to work on the trigger points for you because you may not be able to apply the force needed to release the muscle. Sit on a chair and rest your middle back on the back of the chair. You'll be rounded over a bit; that will allow the trapezius to relax and make it a bit easier to feel for trigger points in supraspinatus. Feel the outside edge of the shoulder blade, the acromion. It's the flat, bony edge at the tip of your shoulder. Follow that bone around to the back

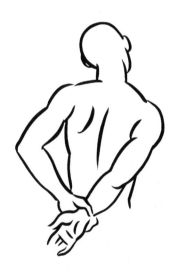

Stretch 1: Supraspinatus

Shoulder Pain

along the spine of the scapula. When you get to the free edge of the bone that is closest to the spine, move your hand up about 1 inch toward the top of your shoulder. Press firmly in that area, enough to get through the trapezius, and you will be able to feel a tight area that is quite sore. You've reached one of the trigger points. Hold that point for a good twenty to thirty seconds and you'll slowly feel it start to release. From there, if you move about 1 inch toward the tip of the shoulder, you should be able to feel another really tight, sore point. Hold and release that one as well.

After working on the muscle, follow up with stretching. Reach behind your back at the level of the waist. Grasp the wrist of the painful arm with your other hand and gently pull the arm across your waist and then up slightly. Hold this position for a count of fifteen to twenty. As your flexibility increases, reach the fingers of that arm up toward the opposite shoulder blade. Strive for full range of motion; your fingers should be able to reach the lower part of your opposite shoulder blade.

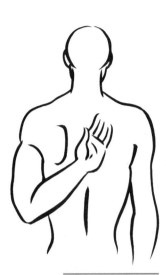

Stretch 2: Supraspinatus

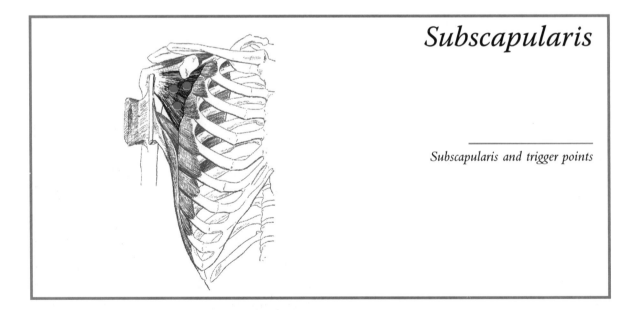

Subscapularis

Subscapularis and trigger points

SUBSCAPULARIS is the muscle most often involved when you have a frozen shoulder. The muscle is a big troublemaker because of its location. Subscapularis is exactly where its name describes—it lies underneath the scapula. To put it another way, subscapularis lies between the shoulder blade and the rib cage. Hence the difficulty in working on it.

Stand with your arms hanging at your sides. Your palms are probably facing your outer thighs. To externally rotate your arm, turn your palms so they face forward. In turning your arms so that your palms move from facing outward to facing toward your thighs again, you would be internally rotating them using subscapularis.

In the worst-case scenario, trigger points in subscapularis cause frozen shoulder—the inability to raise the arm due to both restriction and pain. Pain is usually directly in the back of the shoulder, over the area of the posterior deltoid, and can easily be severe, even when you aren't using the arm. If you have trigger points in subscapularis you may not be able to turn your palm up, and you might even feel pain at the wrist.

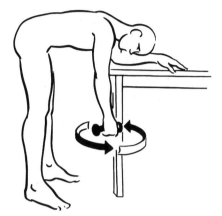

Stretch 1: Subscapularis

Trigger points in subscapularis develop from moments such as catching yourself from falling—something every athlete has done at one time or another. They also develop from actions that require continual internal rotation of the arm, the action the subscapularis is responsible for: swimmers, pitchers, tennis players, and ball players who throw a lot are particularly at risk. Subscapularis might also develop trigger points after the arm is immobilized in a cast or sling for some time, so they might evolve after an injury has healed.

Trigger points in this muscle may be difficult to find and treat, but it is not impossible. Position yourself on a chair with your painful arm hanging between your legs. Reach underneath your arm and locate the sharp outer edge of the shoulder blade. Using your thumb, reach underneath the shoulder blade to find tender, sore points and taut bands of muscle that lie on its inner surface. Once you locate them, hold them for a good fifteen to twenty seconds before moving on to find another.

Try to find tender spots in the muscle lying along the length of the outer edge of the shoulder blade, and then reach under as far as you can to find even more. Remember you are trying to reach in between the shoulder blade and the rib cage to find a muscle that is preventing your shoulder blade, and therefore your arm, from moving away from the rib cage. This will take work and patience and will require many sessions before the muscle returns to its full length.

Follow these sessions with stretches.

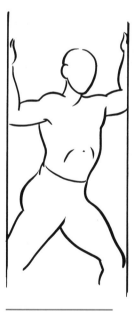

Stretch 2: Subscapularis

1. Bend at the waist so that your upper torso is parallel to the floor and your painful arm is hanging straight down. Grasp a

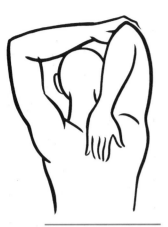

Stretch 3: Subscapularis

heavy weight in your painful arm. Relax and allow gravity to pull the weight toward the floor, stretching subscapularis and moving your shoulder blade along the rib cage. Move your arm in very small circles.

2. Place your arms firmly on each side of a doorway. Stretch the body through the outstretched arms, opening the chest and the shoulders. First place your arms so that your elbows are level with your shoulders. Then extend the arms fully, placing the hands well above your head, or as high up as you can manage.

3. With the elbow bent to 90 degrees, raise the painful arm as high as you can. Draw the forearm back behind the head. Increase the stretch by applying a slight backward pressure just above the elbow.

4. Place your fingers on a wall in front of you. Walk your fingers up the wall as far as you can manage, then turn sideways and do the same thing.

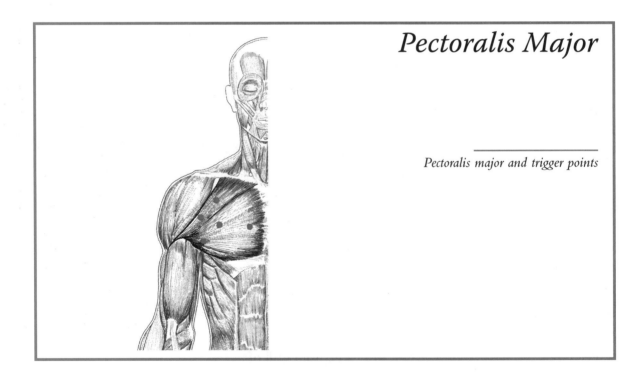

Pectoralis Major

Pectoralis major and trigger points

PECTORALIS MAJOR is the most prominent superficial muscle of the chest. It lies just underneath the breast tissue and can easily be seen contracting by placing your hands on your hips and lightly pressing your hands to your hipbones. Doing this you can see where the fibers of pectoralis major attach to the collarbone, the breastbone (the sternum), and portions of the ribs. The muscle runs obliquely and horizontally across the chest and attaches on the front of the arm near to the lower end of the deltoid.

The action of pectoralis major is to draw the arm toward the chest, an action called adduction, and to medially rotate the arm, turning your palm inward. Because of its location, tightness or restriction of the pectoralis major naturally inhibits movement of the arm and therefore of the shoulder. However, this muscle is frequently overlooked as a source of pain in the shoulder. Excessive tightness of the pectoralis often goes hand in hand with weakness of the upper back muscles, particularly the rhomboids. This produces a round-shouldered appearance, with the shoulders pulled forward. This is not uncommon in weight lifters who overwork the pectorals doing excessive chest presses or flyes. Immobilization of the arm due to a shoulder injury involving other muscles can also be a source of trigger points in the pectorals, as can extended periods of emotional stress and tension.

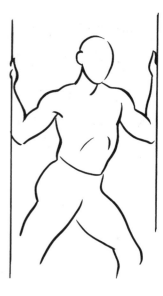

Stretch 1: Pectoralis major

Practicing poor technique in sports that use a rowing motion, such as kayaking, skulling, and canoeing, can lead to trigger points, as can overuse or excessive use of poles while skiing or hiking. Holding on to the handrails instead of allowing the arms to swing naturally when using a treadmill can also restrict the pectorals.

When there are trigger points in pectoralis major, pain radiates to the front of the shoulder, by the anterior deltoid. You may also feel pain in the upper chest, the breast, and possibly the inside of the arm all the way down to the ring finger and pinky. Because of the implications for heart problems associated with chest and arm pain, it is important that you rule out any cardiac involvement before treating yourself for pectoralis trigger points, even if you think that trigger points are the source of the pain. Heart disease can be the source of trigger points in pectoralis major, so check it out to be on the safe side.

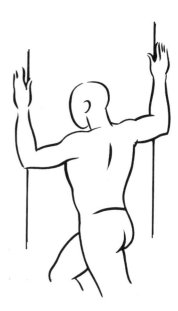

Stretch 2: Pectoralis major

Pectoralis major is the muscle that forms the front wall of the armpit. You can feel for its taut bands and trigger points using a pincer technique. Sit on an armchair and let your elbow rest on the arm piece. There will be a space between your chest and your arm. Reach under the free edge of the armpit with your fingers. You can feel the muscle being lifted off the chest wall a bit. Grasp the upper part of the muscle with your thumb. As you move your thumb across the muscle

Shoulder Pain

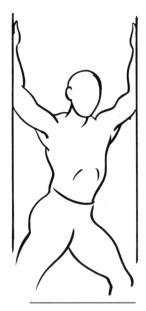

Stretch 3: Pectoralis major

you might feel taut bands of muscle tissue, with tender spots within the taut bands. Use your thumb to press into these spots. You'll feel soreness but it will ease up somewhat as each point lets go.

Work in this way to release tender spots and taut bands throughout pectoralis major and then follow up the muscle release with stretches. The "through the door" stretch will elongate each aspect of the pectoralis. Stand in an open doorway with your forearms placed firmly on the doorjambs. Stretch your body through your outstretched arms, opening your chest and shoulder areas. To stretch the upper fibers of pectoralis major, place your hands at the level of your ears. To stretch the middle fibers of the muscle, place your arms with your elbows level with your shoulders. To stretch the lower fibers of pectoralis, extend your arms fully, well above the level of your head. The stretch that feels the most difficult for you to do is the one you need the most. Concentrate on that one, holding the position for a good count of twenty to thirty.

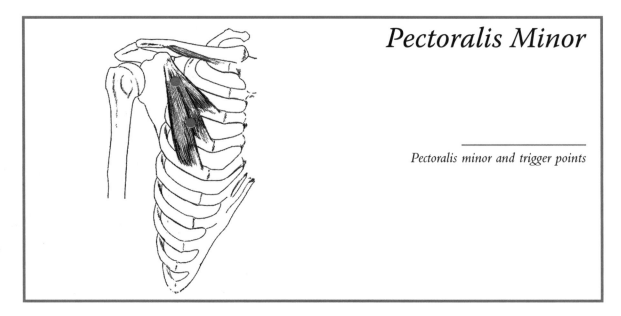

Pectoralis Minor

Pectoralis minor and trigger points

LIKE PECTORALIS MAJOR, PECTORALIS MINOR lies on the chest; but unlike pectoralis major, pectoralis minor acts on the shoulder blade, not the arm. This little muscle lies underneath pectoralis major and attaches to a small bony protrusion on the shoulder blade called the coracoid process. You can feel the coracoid process. Put your fingers on your collarbone (the clavicle), then follow along the clavicle out toward your side. The clavicle first curves outward before it curves inward. When you get to the center of the inward curve, move your hand down about 1 inch. You should be able to feel the hard, bony knob of the coracoid process; it tends to be quite tender to the touch. This is the place of the upper attachment for pectoralis minor. Its other end attaches onto the ribs. The pectoralis minor pulls the shoulder forward and down when it contracts.

Trigger points develop in pectoralis minor in a number of ways, not the least of which is compression. Hikers and backpackers are in danger of developing trigger points when their packs are not fitted properly and weigh heavily on the upper shoulders and chest. Using poles for hiking or skiing can lead to a rounded and stooped upper body posture, which also leads to trigger points in pectoralis minor. Additionally, any activity that brings the shoulder forward, such as nursing an infant, may lead to restriction and trigger points in pectoralis minor.

When trigger points are present the pain is felt just in the front of the shoulder, by anterior deltoid, and possibly in the front of the chest. You might not be able to reach back or forward with your arm at the level of your shoulder. You may also feel pain in the upper chest, the breast, and possibly the inside of the arm all the way down to the ring finger and pinky. Because of the implications for heart problems associated with chest and arm pain, it's important that you rule out any cardiac involvement before treating yourself for pectoralis trigger points, even if you think that that's what the pain is about. Check it out to be on the safe side.

To feel pectoralis minor, sit on a chair with your elbow on the arm of the chair. Position your body so that your elbow is behind your body line. Place your hand on your chest, as though you were saying the Pledge of Allegiance. Your middle finger will probably be just about where the coracoid process is. Now take a deep breath. As you breathe deeply you will feel the contraction of pectoralis minor. Its fibers run obliquely (diagonally) toward the midline of the body. Massage the area deeply as you relax your breath and you'll feel the taut bands of the pectoralis minor with areas of spot tenderness. Hold those tender points.

Stretch pectoralis minor in the same way that you would stretch the upper fibers of pectoralis major. Stand in an open doorway with your forearms placed firmly on the doorjambs. Stretch your body through your outstretched arms, opening your chest and the shoulder area. Place your hands at the level of your ears to best stretch pectoralis minor.

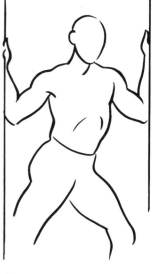

Stretch: Pectoralis minor

Shoulder Pain

Sometimes the action that most strongly creates trigger points in pectoralis minor is breathing high into your chest or holding your breath up in the chest. We're all guilty of doing this, particularly when we're learning a new skill, working hard at the skills we know, or are highly stressed. Once you've released the trigger points in the muscle, work on retraining your breath—breathing deeply into your lower belly rather than up into your chest. See page 173 for the specifics on how to do this.

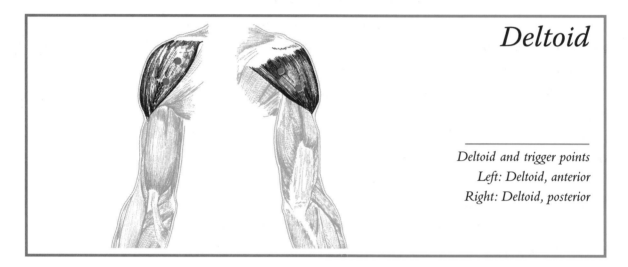

Deltoid

Deltoid and trigger points
Left: Deltoid, anterior
Right: Deltoid, posterior

THE DELTOID MUSCLE gives the shoulder its characteristic shape. The deltoid caps the shoulder. The muscle actually has three sections—the anterior deltoid, the medial deltoid, and the posterior deltoid—each of which works slightly differently from the others. All three aspects of the deltoid are involved in raising the arm and keeping the humerus—the long bone of the upper arm—firmly within the shoulder socket during movement.

The anterior aspect of the deltoid, the one you can see on the front of your shoulder, works with pectoralis major to raise and internally rotate the arm. The medial deltoid raises the arm to the side, while the posterior deltoid, on the back of your shoulder, works with latissimus dorsi and teres major to raise and externally rotate the upper arm. The upper portion of its anterior fibers attach to the outside part of the collarbone; its medial fibers attach to the acromion, the flat, bony edge of the shoulder; and the posterior fibers attach to the spine of the scapula. The lower fibers of all three parts of the deltoid attach about midway down on the humerus onto a bump called the deltoid tuberosity.

Because of its position, deltoid works strongly in any sport that requires overhand, underhand, or sideways arm movement, and therefore is at risk of developing trigger points through overuse. Trigger points also develop in the deltoids as a result of direct trauma—a fall or an impact directly to the upper shoulder—or from a sudden overload that might take place if you have to prevent yourself from falling. If you think about it for a minute, that means that just about any athlete in any sport is at risk for developing trigger points in the deltoid. For those of us who use computers, having the keyboard in a position that is either too low or too high can also lead to trigger points in the deltoid muscle.

The deltoid is second only to infraspinatus as a muscular source of shoulder pain. From a practical standpoint this means that, if you have shoulder pain, after you've checked out infraspinatus you should check out the deltoid. Pain due to trigger points in the deltoid is felt in the front of the shoulder if the trigger points are located in the anterior deltoid and in the back of the shoulder if they are located in the posterior deltoid.

When you have pain from trigger points in the deltoids, your shoulder may feel weak and you may not be able to reach up to the side without pain. The pain is more likely felt when you move rather than when your arm is at rest. This is a good hint. If you have shoulder pain that is felt continuously, both at rest and during motion, it is likely to be coming from a different muscle. Check out the pain pattern images to see what other muscles may be the culprits.

Because the deltoid is so close to the surface of the body, you can easily see and locate this muscle. Use your right hand to feel for trigger points in the left deltoid. First feel your collarbone on your upper chest. Slide your hand under it and out toward your side. Your fingers will end up in a small space where your chest and your shoulder meet; this space is called the deltopectoral groove, because that's where the deltoid muscle meets the pectoralis. The first vertical band of muscle that you feel moving toward the shoulder is the anterior deltoid. Feel within that band of muscle fiber for tight, sore, painful spots. You can press directly on those spots and feel them release—just be patient and relax your shoulder and arm as you work it.

It's much easier to compress the posterior fibers of the deltoid using a tennis ball rather than your hand. Find the trigger points,

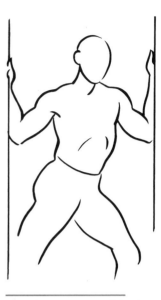

Stretch 1: Anterior deltoid

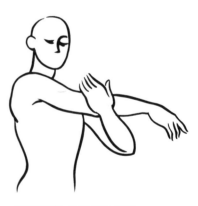

Stretch 2: Posterior deltoid

then lie on the floor and place a tennis ball between you and the floor. Let gravity do its work. All you need to do is to breathe and relax.

Trigger points in the medial deltoid are far less common than trigger points in either the anterior or posterior deltoid. Locate the fibers of the medial deltoid by starting at the acromion, the flat, bony edge of the shoulder. Palpate down from the acromion to identify taut bands and trigger points.

Stretch the anterior deltoid in much the same way you would stretch pectoralis major or subscapularis. Place your arms firmly on each side of a doorway with your hands at the level of your ears. Stretch the body through the outstretched arms, opening the chest and the shoulders. To stretch the posterior deltoid, grasp your arm just above the elbow and pull it across your chest.

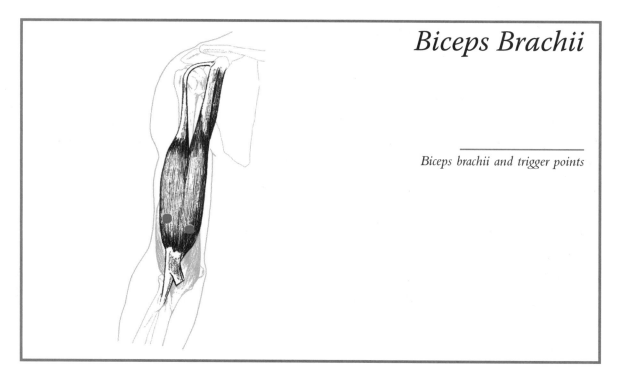

Biceps Brachii

Biceps brachii and trigger points

BICEPS BRACHII forms the familiar bulge on the front of the upper arm. Its upper attachments connect to the upper portions of the shoulder blade and its lower attachment connects to the front of the forearm, just below the elbow. Biceps brachii flexes the forearm and turns the palm upward. It also works with anterior deltoid to flex the upper arm. The biceps is used in any activity that involves bending the arm at the elbow. It is very active during chinning exercises and pull-ups, particularly when the grip faces the body.

Trigger points can develop in the biceps from a chronic or sudden strain caused by heavy lifting—think of climbers or weight lifters overdoing it or dancers practicing lifts over and over again. Carrying a heavily weighted object with the arms outstretched can bring on trigger points. Trigger points can also develop when engaging in any activity that requires that the arm be in a flexed position for some ongoing period of time, such as in playing the guitar or violin.

When trigger points are present in the biceps there is an aching pain in the front of the shoulder that feels close to the surface—it is not a deep pain. There might be some restriction of full extension of the arm. You might not be able to straighten your arm all the way, and your arm may feel somewhat weak. You may have some tenderness in response to pressure over the tendon that attaches the biceps to the forearm at the elbow.

To find the trigger points in the biceps, rest your arm on a table in front of you with your elbow slightly bent. You'll feel a tendon sticking up right at the elbow crease. The tendon will move as you flex and extend your forearm. Moving up from the tendon, massage the muscle first on the outside and then on the inside, feeling for taut bands and the trigger points within them. Trigger points can be found about one-third of the way up the muscle. Once you've found the trigger point hold the point until it begins to soften, and then massage along the taut band.

To stretch the biceps, hold on to a doorjamb with your arm at shoulder level, your elbow straight, and your thumb pointing toward the floor. Turn your body away from the arm, keeping your elbow straight. Hold for a count of fifteen to twenty.

Make sure that you repeat the massage and stretch of the biceps often through the day in order to really release it and keep it released.

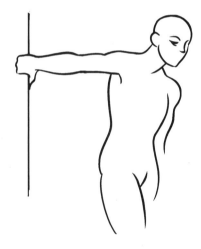

Stretch: Biceps brachii

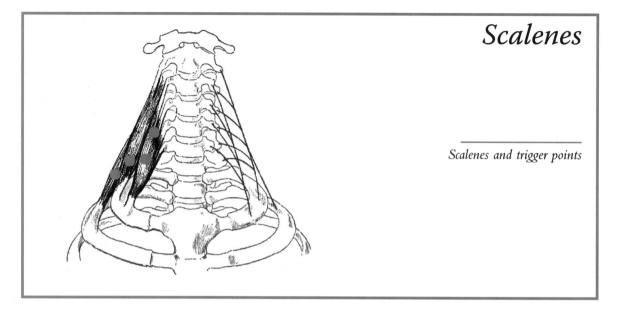

Scalenes

Scalenes and trigger points

THE SCALENES are comprised of three small muscles on the side of the neck that work to bend the neck to the side and to stabilize the neck against sideways impact. Because they attach to the first and second ribs, they are also active in raising the upper rib cage to assist in breathing.

Scalene trigger points are a frequent source of shoulder and arm pain. These small muscles help to support and raise the upper rib cage when carrying, lifting, or pulling heavy objects, particularly with the arms at the level of the waist. Straining to do any of these activities is a source of trigger points. So is carrying the weight of a heavy backpack on the shoulders instead of the hips.

Any kind of force that can produce a whiplash is a source of injury to the scalenes, whether that force is from an automobile accident, a fall, or an impact in contact sports such as football, basketball, or hockey. Breathing high into your chest or holding your breath up in the chest strongly activates the scalenes and can lead to the development of trigger points. We're all guilty of breathing like this, particularly when we're learning a new skill or when we're working hard or feeling highly stressed. Suffering with either chronic or acute breathing problems such as emphysema, pneumonia, bronchitis, or chronic cough can also contribute to the development of trigger points in the scalenes.

Trigger points in the scalenes produce a complex pain pattern that is deep, aching, and persistent. Pain can be experienced in the upper chest and/or the upper back; it can be experienced in the side or back of the shoulder and arm and on the thumb side of the arm and hand, including the thumb and index finger. The pain can be in all of these places or it can be in only one of them, and the location of pain can change from one day to the next. In addition to pain you might feel weakness in the hand and arm that makes you drop things unexpectedly.

The scalenes are often overlooked as the source of these various pain patterns. You can test yourself to see if the scalenes are responsible for your pain. Turn your head fully to the side of your pain and then drop your chin in toward your collarbone. If your pain increases it's a sign that trigger points in the scalenes are causing your pain.

The scalenes are hard to visualize and difficult to feel. Look in the mirror. Tilt your head to the right. As the scalenes contract you'll be able to see the right sternocleidomastoid muscle spanning from underneath your ear to your collarbone. Using your left hand, place the tips of three fingers just behind the sternocleidomastoid at about its midpoint (see page 28) and then straighten your head, keeping your neck relaxed. Press very, very gently back and forth just behind the SCM and you may feel the very thin, taut bands of the scalenes. Once you've found the taut bands try to isolate them under your fingertips, then press very slowly and gently. There are many delicate structures in the front of the neck: you must approach this area with a cautious touch. Even so, once you've found the scalenes you will be able to release them.

Once you've worked on the scalenes, stretching them is essential. Bend your head and neck, aiming the ear of your painless side toward that same shoulder. Hold this position for a count of ten. Then, without changing the angle of your head, rotate your head and face toward the painful side, stretching your cheek toward the ceiling. Hold this position for a count of ten. Return your head and face to the initial position. Now rotate the head and face again, this time aiming your chin for your collarbone. Hold this position for a count of ten before returning it to the initial position. Slowly release your neck from the stretch. You may feel that you are a bit stiffer stretching up rather than stretching down, or vice versa. This tells you which direction needs the most stretch. Remember: these are delicate areas and the stretch, like the touch, has to be gentle. Nonetheless, your work will be effective if you keep at it.

Once you've released the trigger points in the scalenes, work on

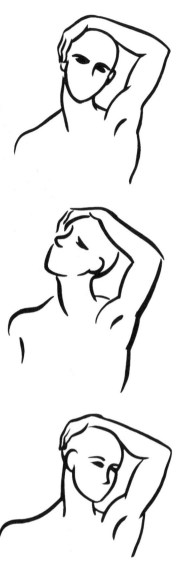

Stretch exercise: Scalenes

retraining your breath, breathing deeply into your lower abdomen rather than up into your chest. See page 173 for the specifics on how to do this.

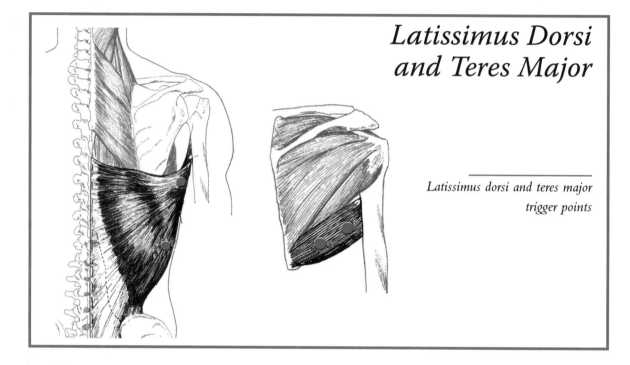

Latissimus Dorsi and Teres Major

Latissimus dorsi and teres major trigger points

LATISSIMUS DORSI is a broad, thin muscle that covers the lower and mid back before it thickens at the level of the armpit. Teres major is a small muscle that lies on the edge of the shoulder blade, just underneath teres minor. Latissimus dorsi twists around teres major and fuses with it before attaching together to the upper arm. Because of the interrelationship between these two muscles, they really have to be considered together. As pectoralis major forms the front wall of the armpit, latissimus dorsi forms its back wall. Latissimus dorsi and teres major work together to bring the arm down and in toward the chest and extend it behind the body line. Think of freestyle swimming. That forward and downward motion is the work of the lats and teres major.

Consider the extent to which these muscles are used in athletics—weight lifting, skiing, hiking, gymnastics, swimming, tennis, basketball, pitching, throwing—the motion of bringing the arm down and in toward the chest is involved in so many sports actions. Trigger points can develop as a function of overusing these muscles in the course of their action or by using them to support a weight with the arms outstretched. Think of the male dancer lifting and holding the apparently weightless ballerina as he carries her across the stage. He is supporting a weight with his arms outstretched, working his lats quite hard as he is doing so.

Trigger points rarely develop in teres major without being present first in latissimus dorsi, but their pain radiates to very different places. The pain associated with latissimus dorsi trigger points is an annoying ache at the bottom of the shoulder blade and surrounding mid back area that neither activity nor rest changes. There might also be pain up to the back of the shoulder and down the inside of the arm, possibly to the ring and little fingers. You may not be able to reach forward and up without pain. The teres major refers pain to the back of the shoulder, by the posterior deltoid area. There might be some pain in the forearm and you may not be able to raise your arm straight above your head, close to your ear.

The most common trigger points in both latissimus dorsi and teres major lie in the muscle mass that forms the back wall of the armpit. Reach under your arm and feel for the sharp outside edge of the shoulder blade. You can use your thumb and fingers to grasp the mass of muscle lying right next to it. That's latissimus dorsi and teres major. Trigger points of teres major can be found on the front side of the back wall of the armpit, 2 to 3 inches above the sharp lower angle of the shoulder blade. You'll be able to deeply massage those with your thumb as you grasp the muscle mass.

The trigger points of latissimus dorsi can be found in that same muscle mass, lower than those of teres major but on the back of the muscle mass. You can massage those with your fingers or you can use a small ball to compress the muscle. Lie on the floor and place the ball between your shoulder blade and the floor. Relax and breathe as you allow gravity to drop your body weight into the ball, compressing the trigger point.

Stretch latissimus dorsi and teres major after you've worked on them. Reach both arms overhead. Grasp the wrist of the hand on the painful side with the opposite hand. Pull the wrist and arm away from the painful side, bending the torso to that side. Hold this position for a count of ten to fifteen.

To stretch teres major, stand (or lie on your back) and raise your arm so that your elbow is close to your ear. Now bend your elbow so your forearm is behind your head. Use your other hand to pull your elbow toward the opposite side.

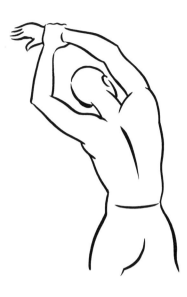

Stretch: Latissimus dorsi and Teres major

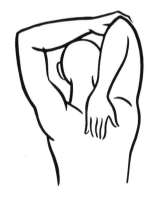

Stretch: Teres major

Shoulder Pain

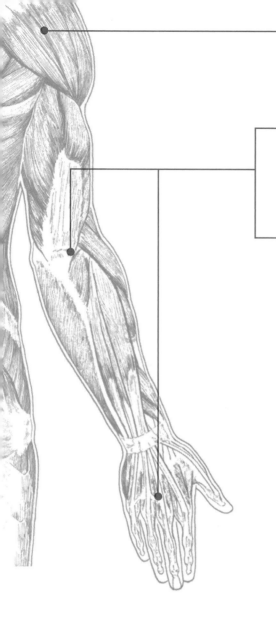

Elbow, Arm, and Hand Pain

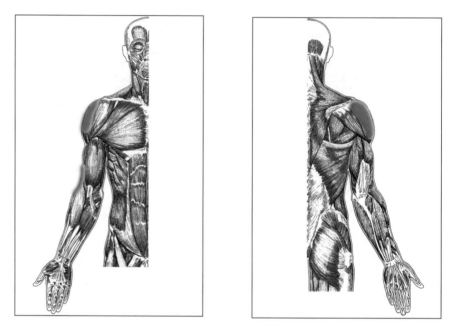

Pain pattern: Supraspinatus

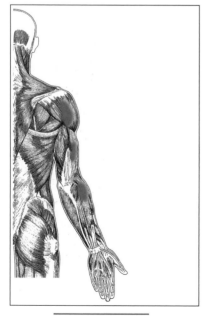

Pain pattern: Triceps brachii

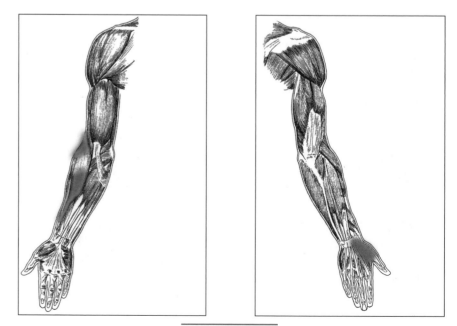

Pain pattern: Brachioradialis

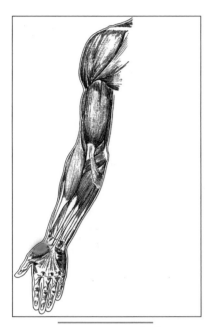

Pain pattern: Brachialis

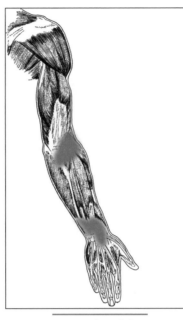

Pain pattern: Hand and finger extensors

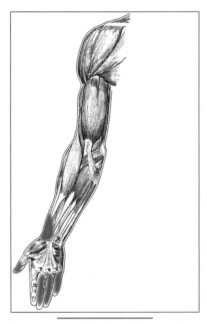

Pain pattern: Hand and finger flexors

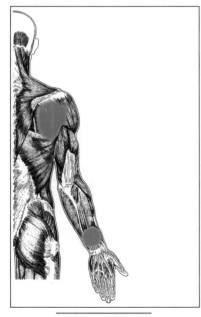

Pain pattern: Subscapularis

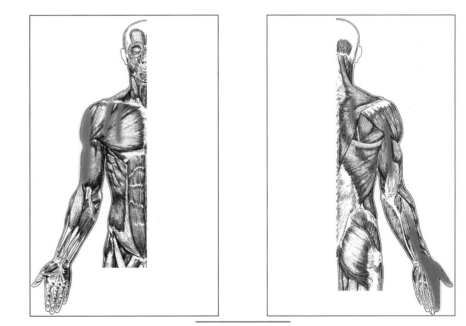

Pain pattern: Scalenes

There are twenty-nine bones that form the structure of the forearm and hand: the two long bones of the forearm, the radius and the ulna; the eight small carpal bones of the wrist; the five metacarpal bones that form the structure of the hand; and the fourteen phalanges that form our fingers. More than two dozen muscles lie on these bones. Together the action of these many bones and muscles of the forearm, wrist, and hand allow us to perform activities that no other species is capable of.

Our ability to use our arms, hands, thumbs, and fingers is one of the major differences between humans and our kin in the animal kingdom. We use our arms, wrists, and hands all day in hundreds of ways and we hardly give it a thought. Our ability to use tools, utensils, and athletic equipment; to write, paint, etch, sculpt, and type, to use our hands in a multitude of ways makes humans capable of things unavailable to members of any other species. Neither these nor the other myriad activities that require the gross- and fine-motor coordination of which the arms and hands are capable would be possible without the miraculous construction of this part of our body.

Because we use our arms, wrists, and hands in almost everything we do, it is possible to sustain an elbow, arm, or hand injury while engaging in almost any sport or endeavor. The possibility is particularly high for those athletes involved in racket sports or in any sport that involves repeated forceful bending and straightening of the arm and/or maintaining a tight grip. An enormous range of athletes fall into this category: tennis, squash, and racquetball players; golfers; hikers or skiers who regularly work with poles; water-skiers; football, baseball, and softball players; rowers, kayakers, and canoers; martial artists who must maintain a tight fist in the performance of their art; and even dancers who hold on to the barre just a bit too intensely. Many athletes and dancers know that passion and excitement can lead to the inadvertent tensing of the muscles. For so many of us this translates into an intense grip.

But athletics is by no means the only arena in which elbow, arm, hand, and finger pain can develop. Think of the gardener who is

> **Cautionary Statement**
>
> Please consult with your physician in the event of any of the following symptoms:
> - an acute injury or intense pain with bleeding or severe bruising
> - joint deformity of the elbow, wrist, or fingers
> - fever, swelling, redness, and /or inability to use the elbow, hand or fingers without pain
> - numbness of the fingers
> - loss of circulation to the hand and fingers resulting in discoloration of the fingers

working the soil in preparation for spring. Digging, turning soil, grasping, lifting, and planting from one- and five-gallon pots—all of this activity works the arms and hands. The office worker, editor, researcher, and anyone who works at a computer throughout the day is clearly at risk for trigger points throughout the arms. The position of the keyboard is often the source of tension in the forearm, wrist, and hand. While often diagnosed as carpal tunnel syndrome, the pain may well be the result of the stresses and strains put upon the musculature of the forearm from computer use. Repetitive strain injuries of the arms and hands are common among people who work in certain industries, particularly those industries involving manufacturing and food production and preparation as well as those of us who work on the body. Massage practitioners, chiropractors, and osteopaths often use pressure techniques that can lead to elbow, wrist, and hand pain. The repeated application of pressure and force can place the muscles of the forearms and hand in awkward and uncomfortable positions and can ultimately injure even those who seek to heal.

The elbow, arms, and hands are often the means by which we play and work. Sometimes we overdo it. Injuries result. Overuse and repetitive strain injuries often lead to the bulk of the muscular pain that we experience. Think about what your actions are part of your sport, your passions, and your work and then consider whether you are one of the many people who has injured an arm or a hand as a function of your activities.

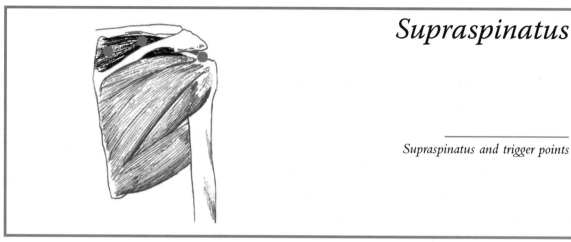

Supraspinatus

Supraspinatus and trigger points

SUPRASPINATUS is a small, thick muscle that lies in the horizontal depression in the upper part of the shoulder blade. Like the other rotator cuff muscles, it attaches to the upper part of the humerus. It lies deep underneath the fibers of the upper trapezius; because of its placement it might be a bit difficult to feel. Like infraspinatus, restrictions in supraspinatus are a common source of shoulder pain.

Trigger points develop in supraspinatus usually in combination with restriction in trapezius and infraspinatus. Carrying something quite heavy with your arms hanging at your side and pulling back against a forward tug are common instigators of trigger points. Rowers and weight lifters are at risk for trigger points at supraspinatus. Pain is usually in the area of the upper shoulder, right by the middle portion of the deltoid. The pain radiates down into the upper arm, sometimes to the forearm and the outside of the elbow. If there are trigger points in supraspinatus you may not be able to reach up to shave or comb your hair or reach back to place your hand into a back pocket or fasten a back button.

Trigger points in supraspinatus are a little difficult to locate because of muscle's location under trapezius. You will most likely need somebody to work on the trigger points for you because you may not be able to apply the force needed to release the muscle. Sit on a chair and rest your middle back on the back of the chair. You'll be rounded over a bit; that will allow the trapezius to relax and make it a bit easier to feel for trigger points in supraspinatus. Feel the outside edge of the shoulder blade, the acromion. It's the flat, bony edge at the tip of your shoulder. Follow that bone around to the back along the spine of the scapula. When you get to the free edge of that bone that is closest to the spine, move your hand up about 1 inch toward the top of your shoulder. Press

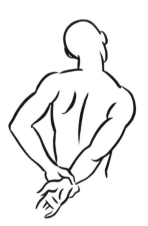

Stretch 1: Supraspinatus

Elbow, Arm, and
Hand Pain

firmly in that area, enough to get through the trapezius, and you will be able to feel a tight area that is quite sore. You've reached one of the trigger points. Hold that point for a good twenty to thirty seconds and you'll slowly feel it start to release. From there, if you move about 1 inch toward the tip of the shoulder, you should be able to feel another really tight, sore point. Hold and release that one as well.

After working on the muscle, follow up with stretching. Reach behind your back at the level of the waist. Grasp the wrist of the painful arm with your other hand and gently pull the arm across your waist and then up slightly. Hold this position for a count of fifteen to twenty. As your flexibility increases, reach the fingers of that arm up toward the opposite shoulder blade. Strive for full range of motion; your fingers should be able to reach the lower part of your opposite shoulder blade.

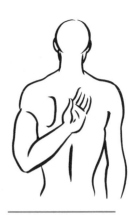

Stretch 2: Supraspinatus

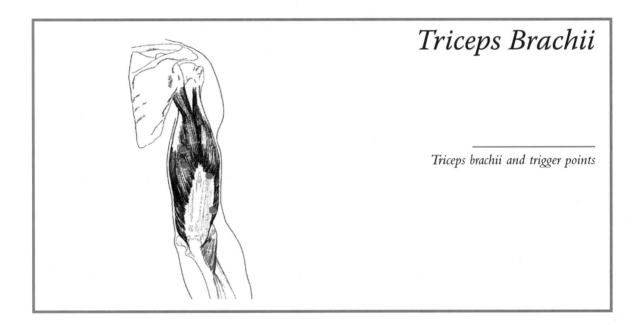

Triceps Brachii

Triceps brachii and trigger points

THE TRICEPS MUSCLE lies on the back of the upper arm. There are three upper attachments that connect to the back of the upper arm and to the shoulder blade. The lower attachment is to the elbow. Triceps extends the elbow, straightening the arm—the triceps works in opposition to the biceps, which flexes the elbow, bending the arm. When the biceps contract to bend the arm, the triceps release; when the triceps contract to extend the elbow, the biceps release. To maintain balanced action it is important to strengthen both the biceps and the triceps when weight training.

Elbow, Arm, and
Hand Pain

■

Trigger points most often develop in the triceps as a result of repeated rapid and forceful bending and straightening of the elbow and pushing heavy objects, such as might take place in weight lifting. The backhand swing and serves in racket sports, the golf swing, pitching in baseball, and long passes in football are examples of this action. When trigger points develop in the triceps pain is felt throughout the back of the upper arm and the lateral epicondyle, the bony outer edge of the elbow. The elbow might be very tender to the touch and the condition might even be diagnosed as epicondylitis, known in lay terms as tennis elbow. Pain may extend through the back of the forearm into the pinky and ring fingers.

Taut bands and trigger points can be found on both the medial (inside) aspect of the triceps muscle and the lateral (outside) aspect. Locate the taut bands by massaging the inside of the triceps with your thumb and the outer side with your fingers. Once you've identified the trigger points, compress them using a small ball. If you lie on the floor and place the ball between your arm and the floor you can use gravity to help to release the muscle.

Stretch triceps by reaching up and back and placing the hand of your painful arm on the upper edge of your shoulder blade, with your elbow as close to your ear as you can get it. Use your non-painful hand to apply pressure just beneath your elbow, directing your upper arm back and in toward your ear.

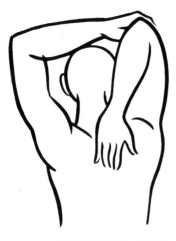

Stretch: Triceps brachii

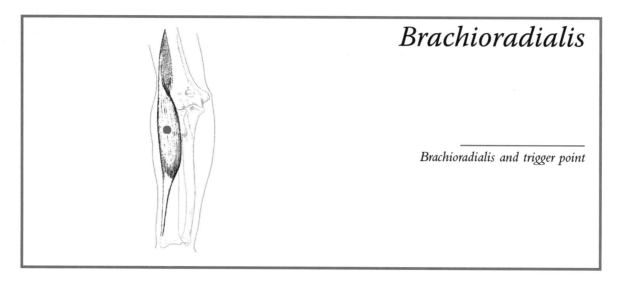

Brachioradialis

Brachioradialis and trigger point

BRACHIORADIALIS gives the forearm its characteristic shape. It is the most superficial muscle of the lateral (thumb side) of the forearm. This muscle is easily identified. Make a light fist and press up against the bottom of a tabletop with the thumb/index finger part of the fist. The brachioradialis becomes clearly prominent. You can feel brachioradialis from its upper attachment on the lower humerus to its lower attachment at the thumb side of the wrist.

Brachioradialis flexes (bends) the forearm at the elbow, especially when the arm is in a neutral position: neither palm down nor palm up. Trigger points develop in brachioradialis due to forceful or repetitive gripping of a large or wide object. Using a tennis racket with a grip that is too wide for your hand is a recipe for the development of trigger points here. When trigger points develop, pain will be felt primarily at the lateral epicondyle—the bony outer side of the elbow—and may extend through the length of the muscle to the web of the thumb on the back of your hand. The pain is often described as tennis elbow. Your grip may feel weak and you may not be able to maintain your grip as reliably as you might like.

Feel for taut bands and trigger points in the upper one-third of the muscle on the front side of your arm. If you grasp the muscle in the upper part of your forearm between your thumb and your fingers, you can use your thumb to feel for ropelike bands with tender spots. When you've found them, hold the trigger point, massage it, and let it release. You may have to do this several times before you feel a release in the muscle. Be patient and work at it.

To stretch brachioradialis, sit on a chair and place your hand palm down, fingers facing toward the back of the chair. Straighten the elbow.

It will do you good to think about the kinds of things that you are doing that led to the development of trigger points. If you do play tennis, check out the grip on your tennis racket to make sure that it suits the size of your hand.

Stretch: Brachioradialis

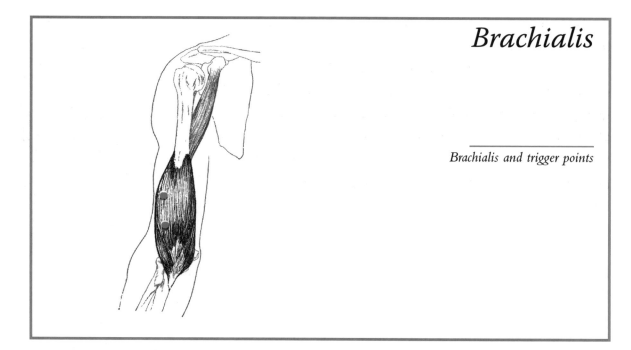

Brachialis

Brachialis and trigger points

WHILE MUCH OF THE CREDIT for forearm flexion is given to biceps brachii, brachialis is actually the primary flexor. This muscle lies underneath the biceps, attaching onto the lower one-half of the humerus at its upper end and to the ulna on its lower end. Brachialis is your "chinning" muscle. When your palms are facing you on a chinning bar, brachialis is the workhorse.

Trigger points develop in brachialis primarily as a function of overloading the muscle. An overload can occur by placing too much weight on the muscle repetitively or continuously. Carrying heavy loads with the elbows bent, chinning, and weight lifting are all examples of actions that can affect this muscle. When trigger points are present, pain and tenderness will be experienced at the base of the thumb in both the front and the back of the hand. The pain may be increased when you use your hand and your thumb.

Because of its position underneath the biceps, you will have to move the bulk of the biceps out of the way in order to locate brachialis. Place your elbow on the arm of a chair or a low table with your palm down. Flex your arm about 30 degrees to relax the biceps. Use the pads of your fingers to move biceps brachii medially toward your body. You can then palpate brachialis in the lower one-half of the upper arm. It's a thick muscle, so when you find taut bands and the trigger points contained within them you'll have to press deeply into the muscle in order to release the trigger points. Hold each area of tightness for twenty to thirty seconds before you

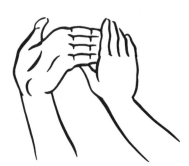

Stretch 1: Brachialis

Elbow, Arm, and
Hand Pain

82

release and massage it. Return to it as often as you can in order to release it completely.

After working on the muscle, stretch it by extending the arm out in front of you with the elbow fully straightened. Pull back gently on the hand and fingers to increase the stretch. You can also place the hand beside your seated body, palm down and the fingers pointing back. This will markedly increase the stretch. Hold the position for a count of ten to fifteen. Repeat several times throughout the day.

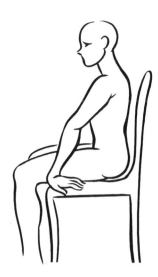

Stretch 2: Brachialis

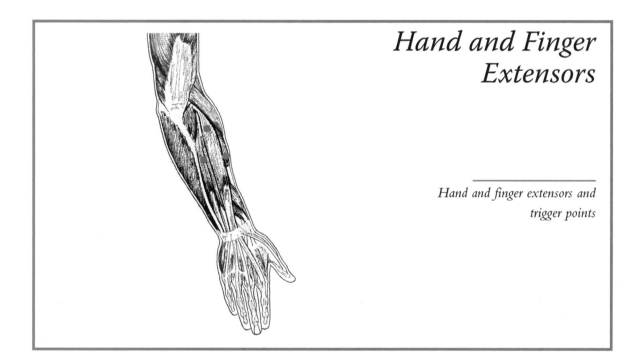

Hand and Finger Extensors

Hand and finger extensors and trigger points

THE HAND EXTENSORS are comprised of numerous small muscles that lie on the back of the forearm. They attach via a single common tendon to the lateral epicondyle of the humerus, the bony outside edge of the elbow. This tendon is the site of the inflammation syndrome known as lateral epicondylitis, the infamous "tennis elbow." The lower attachments of the hand extensors are to several of the metacarpal bones of the hand, the long bones that connect the wrist to the fingers.

These muscles work as a group to extend the wrist, bending

Elbow, Arm, and
Hand Pain

it back. Pain and tenderness that result from trigger points in the hand extensors is often diagnosed as tennis elbow. The pain can radiate throughout the back of the forearm and into the back of the wrist. The outside edge of the elbow, the lateral epicondyle, can be extremely tender to the touch. A weak and unreliable grip is a symptom often associated with the pain. No wonder trigger point involvement here is so frequently diagnosed as tennis elbow! Sufferers often take anti-inflammatory medications to try to deal with the pain and yet, because the muscles are not being addressed, this treatment is frequently unsuccessful at providing relief.

A repetitive or forceful grip is generally the source of trigger points in the hand extensors. Think of the type of sports that involve maintaining a handgrip; these are the athletes that are most at risk for forearm muscle injury. They include tennis players or players of any racket sports, golfers, baseball or softball players, snow- and water-skiers, hikers who use poles, and weight lifters.

A detailed understanding of the specific muscles involved is not really necessary for their release using manual pressure techniques. Locate the taut bands and trigger points on the back of the forearm. You'll get a clear idea of the layout of each of the muscles on the arm by extending (bending backward) each finger and your wrist while you are massaging your arm. Massage each of the muscles from its upper to its lower attachment. You'll be able to identify the tender points. Once you've located them, hold them without too much pressure and flex your hand at the same time (bending it toward your palm). The gentle stretch that you apply by flexing your hand will help the muscle to release. It's really important that you keep at this to completely release the muscles.

Follow treatment with even more stretch. Extend your elbow out in front of you with your palm up and then flex your wrist. Aim the tip of your middle finger for the front of your forearm for the greatest stretch. You can also sit on a chair. While keeping your elbow straight, place the back of your hand on the seat beside you, palm up, to stretch the back of the forearm.

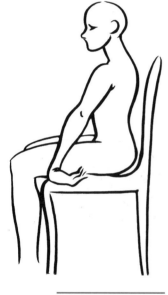

Stretch: Hand and finger extensors

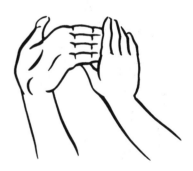

Hand and Finger Flexors

Hand and finger flexors and trigger points

THE HAND AND FINGER FLEXORS are comprised of numerous small muscles that lie on the front of the forearm. They attach via a single common tendon to the medial epicondyle of the humerus, the bony inside edge of the elbow. Their lower attachments are to each finger. As a group they work to flex the hand, the wrist, and the fingers.

Trigger points develop in the hand and finger flexors as a result of repetitive or prolonged gripping, twisting, or pulling movements of the hand and fingers. Think of the type of sports that involve gripping; these are the athletes that are at risk for forearm muscle injury. They include tennis players or players of any racket sports, golfers, baseball or softball players, snow- and water-skiers, hikers who use poles, and weight lifters. Boxers or martial arts practitioners are subject to restrictions of the forearm flexors because of the strength with which they seek to maintain a tight fist. When there are trigger points in these muscles pain is felt in the fingers and at the front of the wrist, just above the thumb. A trigger finger may also develop; trigger finger is the inability to straighten the finger without a snapping or a clicking at the joint.

A detailed understanding of the specific muscles involved really is not necessary for their release using manual pressure techniques. Locate the taut bands and trigger points on the front of the forearm.

Stretch 1: Hand and finger flexors

Elbow, Arm, and
Hand Pain

■

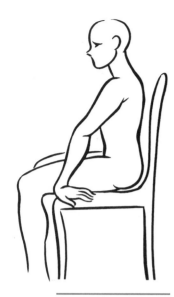

Stretch 2: Hand and finger flexors

You'll get a clear idea of the layout of each of the muscles on the arm by flexing each finger and your wrist (bending them toward the palm) while you are massaging your arm. Massage each muscle from its upper to its lower attachment; you'll be able to identify the tender points. Once you've located them, hold them without too much pressure and extend your wrist (bend it back) at the same time. The gentle stretch that you apply by bending your wrist back will help the muscle to release. It's really important that you keep at this to completely release the muscles.

Follow treatment with even more stretch. With your elbow straight, slowly press the fingers and the wrist into extension, bending the wrist back using your opposite hand. Pressing your palm and your fingers onto a flat surface will also stretch the flexors. Hold the position for a good count of five to ten; repeat it often throughout the day for a complete release.

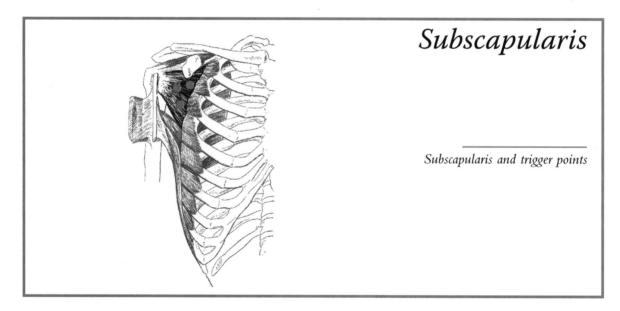

Subscapularis

Subscapularis and trigger points

SUBSCAPULARIS is the muscle most often involved when you have a frozen shoulder. The muscle is a big troublemaker because of its location. Subscapularis is exactly where its name describes—it lies underneath the scapula. To put it another way, subscapularis lies between the shoulder blade and the rib cage. Hence the difficulty in working on it.

In the worst-case scenario, trigger points in subscapularis cause frozen shoulder—the inability to raise the arm due to both restriction and pain. Pain is usually directly in the back of the shoulder, over the area of the posterior deltoid, and can easily be severe, even when you aren't using the arm. If you have trigger points in subscapularis

Elbow, Arm, and
Hand Pain

you may not be able to turn your palm up, and you might even feel pain at the wrist.

Trigger points in subscapularis develop from moments such as catching yourself from falling—something every athlete has done at one time or another. They also develop from actions that require continual internal rotation of the arm, the action the subscapularis is responsible for: swimmers, pitchers, tennis players, and ball players who throw a lot are particularly at risk. Subscapularis might also develop trigger points after the arm is immobilized in a cast or sling for some time, so they might evolve after an injury has healed.

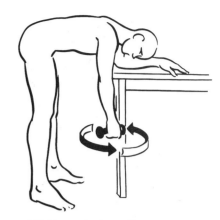

Stretch 1: Subscapularis

Trigger points in this muscle may be difficult to find and treat, but it is not impossible. Position yourself on a chair with your painful arm hanging between your legs. Reach underneath your arm and locate the sharp outer edge of the shoulder blade. Using your thumb, reach underneath the shoulder blade to find tender, sore points and taut bands of muscle that lie on its inner surface. Once you locate them, hold them for a good fifteen to twenty seconds before moving on to find another.

Try to find tender spots in the muscle lying along the length of the outer edge of the shoulder blade, and then reach under as far as you can to find even more. Remember you are trying to reach in between the shoulder blade and the rib cage to find a muscle that is preventing your shoulder blade, and therefore your arm, from moving away from the rib cage. This will take work and patience and will require many sessions before the muscle returns to its full length.

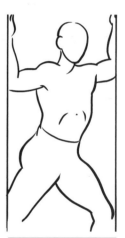

Stretch 2: Subscapularis

Follow these sessions with stretches.

1. Bend at the waist so that your upper torso is parallel to the floor and your painful arm is hanging straight down. Grasp a heavy weight in your painful arm. Relax and allow gravity to pull the weight toward the floor, stretching subscapularis and moving your shoulder blade along the rib cage. Move your arm in very small circles.

2. Place your arms firmly on each side of a doorway. Stretch the body through the outstretched arms, opening the chest and the shoulders. First place your arms so that your elbows are level with your shoulders. Then extend the arms fully, placing the hands well above your head, or as high up as you can manage.

3. With the elbow bent to 90 degrees, raise the painful arm as high as you can. Draw the forearm back behind the head. Increase

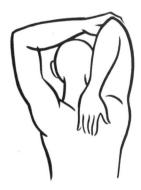

Stretch 3: Subscapularis

Elbow, Arm, and
Hand Pain

the stretch by applying a slight backward pressure just above the elbow.

4. Place your fingers on a wall in front of you. Walk your fingers up the wall as far as you can manage, then turn sideways and do the same thing.

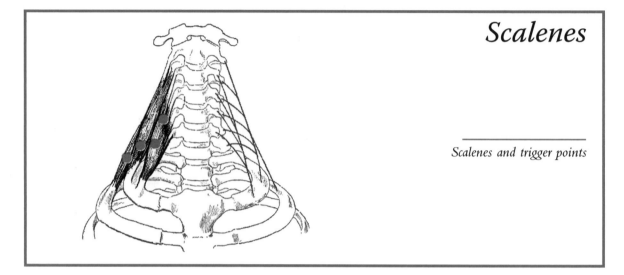

Scalenes

Scalenes and trigger points

THE SCALENES are comprised of three small muscles on the side of the neck that work to bend the neck to the side and to stabilize the neck against sideways impact. Because they attach to the first and second ribs, they are also active in raising the upper rib cage to assist in breathing.

Scalene trigger points are a frequent source of shoulder and arm pain. These small muscles help to support and raise the upper rib cage when carrying, lifting, or pulling heavy objects, particularly with the arms at the level of the waist. Straining to do any of these activities is a source of trigger points. So is carrying the weight of a heavy backpack on the shoulders instead of the hips.

Any force that can produce a whiplash is a source of injury to the scalenes, whether that force is from an automobile accident, a fall, or an impact in contact sports such as football, basketball, or hockey. Breathing high into your chest or holding your breath up in the chest strongly activates the scalenes and can lead to the development of trigger points. We're all guilty of breathing like this, particularly when we're learning a new skill or when we're working hard or feeling highly stressed. Suffering with either chronic or acute breathing problems such as emphysema, pneumonia, bronchitis, or chronic cough can also contribute to the development of trigger points in the scalenes.

Trigger points in the scalenes produce a complex pain pattern that is deep, aching, and persistent. Pain can be experienced in the upper chest and/or the upper back; it can be experienced in the side or back of the shoulder and arm and on the thumb side of the arm and hand, including the thumb and index finger. The pain can be in all of these places or it can be in only one of them, and the location of pain can change from one day to the next. In addition to pain you might feel weakness in the hand and arm that makes you drop things unexpectedly.

The scalenes are often overlooked as the source of these various pain patterns. You can test yourself to see if the scalenes are responsible for your pain. Turn your head fully to the side of your pain and then drop your chin in toward your collarbone. If your pain increases it's a sign that trigger points in the scalenes are causing your pain.

The scalenes are hard to visualize and difficult to feel. Look in the mirror. Tilt your head to the right. As the scalenes contract you'll be able to see the right sternocleidomastoid muscle spanning from underneath your ear to your collarbone. Using your left hand, place the tips of three fingers just behind the sternocleidomastoid at about its midpoint (see page 28) and then straighten your head while keeping your neck relaxed. Press very, very gently back and forth just behind the SCM and you may feel the very thin, taut bands of the scalenes. Once you've found the taut bands try to isolate them under your fingertips, then press very slowly and gently. There are many delicate structures in the front of the neck: you must approach this area with a cautious touch. Even so, once you've found the scalenes you will be able to release them.

Once you've worked on the scalenes, stretching them is essential. Bend your head and neck, aiming the ear of your painless side toward that same shoulder. Hold this position for a count of ten. Then, without changing the angle of your head, rotate your head and face toward the painful side, stretching your cheek toward the ceiling. Hold this position for a count of ten. Return your head and face to the initial position. Now rotate the head and face again, this time aiming your chin for your collarbone. Hold this position for a count of ten before returning it to the initial position. Slowly release your neck from the stretch. You may feel that you are a bit stiffer stretching up rather than stretching down, or vice versa. This tells you which direction needs the most stretch. Remember: these are delicate areas and the stretch, like the touch, has to be gentle. Nonetheless, your work will be effective if you keep at it.

Once you've released the trigger points in the scalenes, work on retraining your breath, breathing deeply into your lower abdomen rather than up into your chest. See page 173 for the specifics on how to do this.

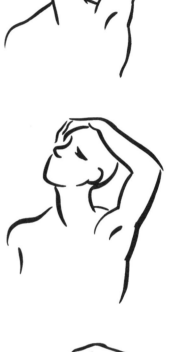

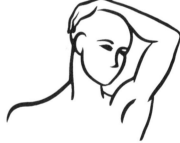

Stretch: Scalenes

Elbow, Arm, and
Hand Pain

■

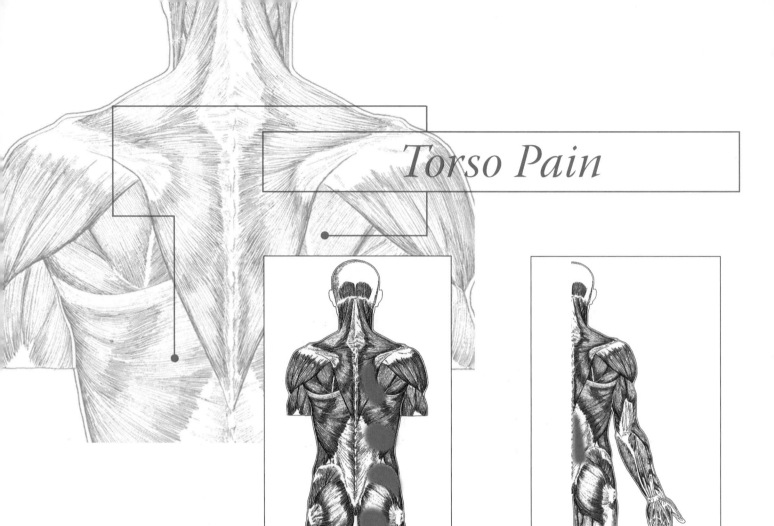

Torso Pain

Pain pattern: Erector spinae

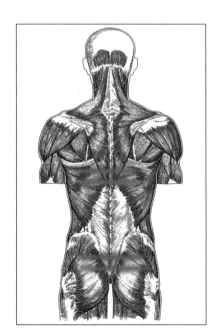

Pain pattern: Iliopsoas

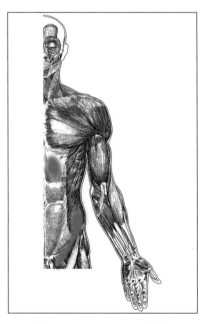

Transversus abdominis, Internal
oblique, External oblique

Pain pattern: The Abdominals

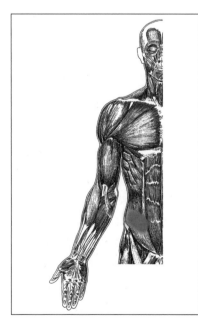

Rectus abdominis

Pain pattern: The Abdominals

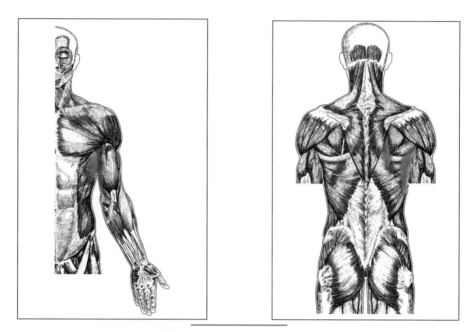

Pain pattern: Serratus anterior

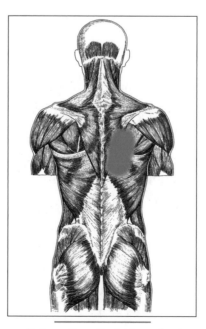

Pain pattern: Latissimus dorsi

Every athlete and dancer understands the critical importance of developing strength in the muscles of the torso: the abdominal and back muscles. These muscles are so essential to the effective practice of technique that a complete system of exercise was developed for the purpose of truly making our core, our center, the focal point from which we move.

In the early decades of the twentieth century, Joseph Pilates developed a practice that has come to be known simply by his name: Pilates. It is based on the notion that when the muscles of the core, "the powerhouse" of the body, are working properly, balanced physical, mental, and spiritual well-being ensue. Joseph Pilates believed that through concentration, control, precision, flowing movement, and proper breathing the integration of mind and body would occur. These are the principles of action upon which the Pilates method was founded.

Pilates was extensively practiced by famously successful dancers in the mid-1900s, including George Ballanchine, Hanya Holm, and others, and in the past twenty years has become increasingly well-known. Pilates is practiced by athletes, dancers, and seekers of health and well-being throughout the world. An interesting by-product of the correct practice of Joseph Pilates' method is the positive influence it has on the practice of any physical endeavor. It became obvious that sport and dance practice would improve by strengthening the core, because the force generated in the large muscles of the legs could be evenly transferred to the upper shoulders and arms through a stable trunk.

The groups of muscles that support the trunk are the focus of this practice. These are the abdominal muscles; the paraspinal muscles of the back, the erector spinae; and quadratus lumborum and iliopsoas, the muscles of the posterior abdominal wall. Their combined actions provide all movements that take place in the trunk. The erector spinae group extends the spine and keeps the spine erect (hence the name). The abdominals work with quadratus lumborum to rotate the spine and to bend the torso to the side (lateral bending), and the rectus abdominis works with iliopsoas to flex the trunk (bend it forward). The strength and suppleness of these muscles allow for the pelvic and spinal stability that contribute to postural integrity, improved balance, efficient movement, and organ support. The reflection of these results is optimal function and a vibrant physicality.

Unfortunately the converse is equally true. When the muscles of the abdomen and torso are weak, the stability of the spine and pelvis and the functioning of the organs contained by these muscles are compromised. It is with these muscles that we see the clear connection between muscular integrity and organ function—between strength and health. It is particularly important to respect this connection as we move into our older years.

Injuries to the back muscles can occur in almost any sport or endeavor, particularly those activities that involve forward bending and twisting, such as tennis, golf, football, bowling, dance, and gymnastics. One of the most common sources of injury is poor muscle conditioning or an inadequate warm-up. The golfer who plays eighteen holes of golf on the first warm Sunday in spring after spending the winter on the couch is vying for a back injury. So is the avid gardener who decides that the entire garden needs to be readied for planting in one weekend. Unprepared for the degree of work that is required in a round of golf or a day of raking and digging, the back muscles become easily strained through overload and overuse. Improper lifting can also lead to overload of the paraspinal muscles and the development of trigger points.

Immobility can be as damaging to the musculature as overuse. Sitting for hours on a plane, in a car, or at a desk can easily lead to trigger points and subsequent weakness and stiffness in the musculature of the back.

So many of us ricochet from one end of the spectrum to the other: overuse on the weekends to immobility during the week. Movement is yet another area in which we must work to create balance for the good of our overall health.

Injuries to the abdominal musculature take place during sports, dance, gymnastics, hatha yoga, Pilates practice, and many everyday activities. These injuries often occur due to overstretching or overexertion. Strenuous lifting can be a source of abdominal strain because it requires that the abdominal musculature engage to fix the upper part of the torso to perform the action. Many athletes work out at the gym to strengthen their musculature. Overdoing abdominal workouts in intensity or frequency and workouts that involve heavy lifting can be a source of strain within the musculature.

It's important to be aware that if you have been recently pregnant or if your abdominal muscles are otherwise overstretched and have poor tone, your muscles may sustain injuries and the spinal vertebrae of your lower back (the lumbar spine) may be subject to alignment problems or dysfunction related to the spinal column. Your torso and spine depend on the strength of your abdominal muscles for support, movement, and organ containment; weakness in the musculature requires that your muscles work much harder to accomplish this already complex job. It's important to strengthen your abs, but if you're just beginning be careful, be patient, and build up slowly.

Many of the symptoms associated with trigger points in the abdominal muscles are related to dysfunction of the digestive and genitourinary organs (the stomach, small intestine, large intestine, bladder, ovaries, uterus, and testes). Symptoms may include heartburn, bloating, indigestion, vomiting, cramps, dysmenorrhea, and urinary frequency or retention. Even if you believe that your symptoms are related to abdominal trigger points, it is important to rule out organic disease or dysfunction. See your physician for a medical evaluation prior to self-treatment. If your pain is severe and is accompanied by fever or abdominal rigidity or bleeding, see your physician immediately.

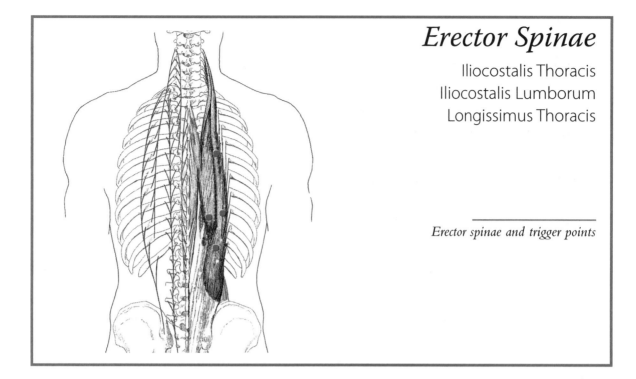

Erector Spinae

Iliocostalis Thoracis
Iliocostalis Lumborum
Longissimus Thoracis

Erector spinae and trigger points

THE ERECTOR SPINAE GROUP is the most superficial of the paraspinal muscles, muscles that lie on either side of the spine. This group of muscles is considered to be the "true" back muscles. The function of erector spinae is to maintain upright posture and to move and protect the spinal column.

Erector spinae extends from a single broad attachment at the sacrum, the upper part of the pelvis, and each of the five lumbar vertebrae in the low back upward to each of the ribs and the vertebrae adjacent to them, the thoracic vertebrae. When these muscles work bilaterally they straighten the back and extend the spine; when only one side is in action they work with the abdominals to bend the torso to the side.

The most common source of trigger points in erector spinae is from overloading the muscles through straining while lifting improperly. Bending forward from the hips to lift an object from the floor, rather than reaching from bent knees, places a excessive load on these muscles. Straining to have a bowel movement and coughing also produce a strong contraction of erector spinae. The erector spinae is in a continual state of contraction in the person who has a strongly arched low back. This chronic overload may lead to trigger points. Immobility can also lead to trigger points in erector spinae: sitting for extended periods of time without break can cause trigger points to develop. Whether sitting at a desk or on an airplane, it's important to move around at regular intervals to prevent restriction of erector spinae.

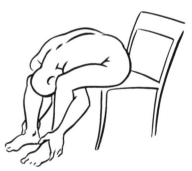

Stretch 1: Erector spinae

Torso Pain

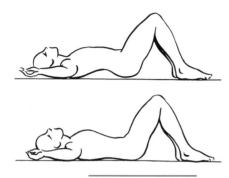

Stretch 2: Erector spinae

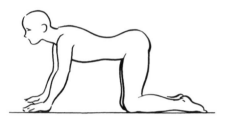

Stretch 3: Erector spinae

Trigger points can develop at just about any level of the muscle. The pain that is produced can be either close to the trigger point or referred farther from the trigger point, along the course of the muscle. Trigger points in the low back portion of erector spinae tend to refer pain to the low back and buttocks; trigger points in the rib cage portion of the muscle tend to refer pain upward, higher in the back. Some trigger points even produce pain in both the back and the front of the torso. Pain is frequently accompanied by restricted motion. Both forward bending and sidebending may be uncomfortable. If trigger points are present in both sides of erector spinae at the level of your lowest rib, you might not be able to get out of a chair or climb stairs comfortably.

The easiest way to treat your own trigger points is to lie on a tennis ball. You can make a convenient treatment device by placing two tennis balls in a sock and tying the sock so the balls stay together. Lie on the floor and place the balls, one on each side of the spine, at the level of the trigger point. Relax and just let gravity do its work. Breathing deeply helps to relax the muscle. Each time you exhale, allow your body to drop down further onto the balls. Stay at one point for several minutes and then move the balls to another level of the spine. It may take some time but the muscle will slowly relax.

Follow up with stretches. Do any one that you can manage, and then work up to the other two.

1. Sit comfortably on a chair with your feet placed flat on the floor. Fold your torso toward the floor, reaching forward and down with your arms. A key here is to allow your head and neck to drop down and hang loosely. Hold this position for a count of twenty to thirty. Slowly lift back up to a seated position.
2. Lie on your back. Bend your knees and place the soles of your feet on the floor. Exhale and slowly drop your low back toward the floor. Hold for a count of five and then release. Repeat this several times, making sure that you aren't pulling your belly in and tucking your pelvis.
3. Position your body on your hands and knees. Arch your back, lifting both your head and your buttocks toward the ceiling. Hold this position for a count of five. Then round your back, aiming your head and your tailbone for the floor. Hold again for a count of five. Alternate these two movements three to four times.

Following treatment and stretches, use a moist heating pad or take a hot bath to hydrate the muscle. It will help enormously! If you're using a moist heating pad, lie on your belly and place a pillow underneath your ankles. This will put a bend in your knees and help to take pressure off the low back.

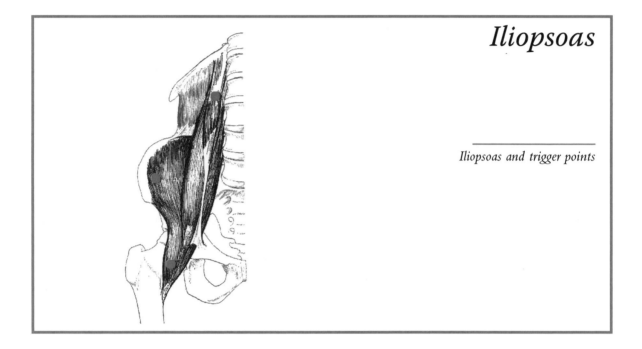

Iliopsoas

Iliopsoas and trigger points

ILIOPSOAS is the primary flexor of the trunk and the most powerful of the thigh flexors. Iliopsoas, often referred to simply as "the psoas," is comprised of two and sometimes three muscles: the psoas, which lies beside the lumbar vertebrae; the iliacus, which lines the inner part of the crests of the pelvis; and psoas minor, which lies in front of psoas major. (Psoas minor is absent in approximately 40 percent of the population.)

Iliopsoas lies on the inside (the front part) of the spine, behind the abdominal organs. It attaches to the sides of the lumbar vertebrae in the low back and to the inside of the pelvis. It passes underneath the inguinal ligament in the groin and attaches to the upper part of the femur, the long bone of the thigh. When the legs are fixed, the contraction of iliopsoas results in bending forward at the hips (flexion of the trunk); when the legs are free, its contraction results in bringing the knee toward the chest (flexion of the thigh on the hip).

Iliopsoas functions in maintaining our upright posture. It works continuously during walking and is considerably active during jogging, running, and kicking. It is highly active during the last 60 degrees of a sit-up. Like the other muscles of the torso, its significance in athletics and dance cannot be emphasized enough.

Trigger points develop in iliopsoas through overload. A repetitive overload would be the repeated forceful flexion of the hip that takes place in dance, gymnastics, jogging, running, hurdling, and sports that involve high kicks—such as those performed by football field kickers. Doing an excessive numbers of sit-ups could also result in trigger points in this muscle for the same reason. A sustained overload would be sitting for extended periods of time with your knees higher than your hips or lying in the fetal position for extended periods without moving.

When trigger points are present in the upper part of iliopsoas, pain is referred in a vertical pattern alongside the vertebrae of the low back. The pain will be on one side only, the side of the affected muscle. Pain will be much worse while you're standing and will be alleviated when you lie down with your hips and knees bent. When there are trigger points in the lower parts of iliopsoas, pain will be felt in the groin and the front of the upper thigh. A severely restricted iliopsoas will prevent you from standing upright.

Palpating iliopsoas is difficult but not impossible. To find the upper part of iliopsoas, lie on your back. Bend your knees and place your feet on the floor. Shift both knees to the side, *away* from your pain. By lying this way you'll be able to reach beneath some of the abdominal contents to work on iliopsoas. Place your hands at the level of your navel and then shift them a couple of inches to the side, to the outer border of the rectus abdominis (page 102). Press straight down and in toward the midline of your body to palpate taut bands of iliopsoas. Taut bands might feel sore and ropelike. Press deeply along the length of the band from the area just underneath your navel to the inguinal ligament.

Lie on your back with your knees up to palpate trigger points along the inside of the rim of the pelvis. This time you won't have to drop your knees to the side. Find your inguinal ligament at your groin (see the instructions at Adductors, page 130). Trace the inguinal ligament upward toward its attachment on the pelvis, your hip bone. Cup your fingers around the bone, trying as best you can to press straight down and then into the inside rim with your fingertips. You'll find trigger points there that refer pain into your groin. You can also release iliopsoas trigger points by applying direct pressure to the portion of the inguinal ligament that is closest to the hip bone.

To find the trigger point that refers pain into the front of your thigh, you'll need to locate the femoral triangle (page 131). Iliopsoas taut bands can be palpated on the outer side of the floor of the femoral triangle. Press gently into the area to release the trigger point. Remember that there are many delicate structures within that triangle, so be sure to exercise care when you compress that region.

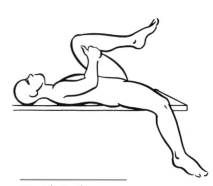

Stretch 1: Iliopsoas

As with all muscles, stretching is necessary to obtain complete release. Lie on the edge of a bed or table and let the leg of your painful side hang off the end. Flex the thigh and leg of your other side to keep your pelvis flat on the table. Let gravity work to stretch the leg down toward the floor. Hold this position for a count of twenty to thirty.

You can stretch iliopsoas by lying on the floor on your abdomen. Place your hands, palms down, next to your chest. Raise your upper body, supporting it by keeping your weight on your arms. Arch your head and neck toward the ceiling; keep your hips, legs, and feet relaxed on the floor. Hold the stretch for a count of twenty to thirty. Release the stretch by relaxing your arms and bending your elbows to slowly bring your body down to the starting position.

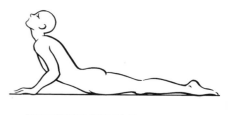

Stretch 2: Iliopsoas

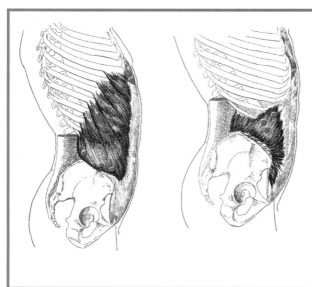

The Abdominals

Transversus Abdominis
External Oblique
Internal Oblique

Abdominals and trigger points
Left: External oblique
Right: Internal oblique

THE ABDOMINAL MUSCLES—transversus abdominis, internal oblique, external oblique, and rectus abdominis—lie on the front and sides of the torso. Together with the muscles of the posterior abdominal

Torso Pain

wall—the quadratus lumborum and iliopsoas—they form a sheath, a pocket, that contains many of the major organs of the body and the tissues that connect them. The liver, gall bladder, stomach, small intestine, large intestine, spleen, pancreas, and kidneys lie within this sheath. The sides and part of the front of the sheath are formed by transversus abdominis and the internal and external oblique. The midline of the sheath is formed by rectus abdominis and back of the sheath is formed by the psoas muscle and quadratus lumborum. The diaphragm forms the upper boundary of the sheath. These muscles, working together with the diaphragm, aid organ function by providing support, protection, and compression during activity and respiration. The abdominal muscles are layered and their differing fiber directions produce the various motions that the torso is capable of.

Transversus abdominis is the deepest of the four abdominal muscles. Its fibers run almost horizontally, back to front, attaching in the back to the lumbar vertebrae through a broad, flat tendon and on the sides to the lower half of the rib cage and the upper part of the pelvis. It attaches in the front of the body at the pubic bone and to what is called the linea alba, the vertical midline tendon that connects all the abdominal muscles. (This is the midline depression in the coveted "six-pack," the physical presentation when the abs are really developed.)

The internal oblique lies just superficial to (on top of) transversus. Its fibers attach at the linea alba and run obliquely toward the outside of the body to connect to the upper part of the pelvis and the lower ribs. External oblique is the most superficial muscle on the side of the body. Its fibers run obliquely toward the midline. (If you place your hand in the pocket of a baseball jacket, your fingers would approximate the fiber direction of external oblique.) External oblique connects the front part of the lower half of the rib cage and the linea alba.

The transversus and the obliques work together to compress the abdomen and to rotate and bend the trunk to the side. When you "pull your navel toward your spine," as you're instructed when doing core work or Pilates work, you are using transversus. When you are doing oblique crunches, bringing your elbow to the opposite knee, external and internal oblique are the muscles that you are using to rotate and bend your torso to the side.

Trigger points can develop in the obliques from overuse or strain.

Vigorous or sustained twisting of the torso falls into that category. So does the considerable muscular forces that are experienced during childbirth. Trigger points may develop in the presence of dysfunction or disease of the abdominal organs, abdominal surgery, or abdominal surgical scars. Poor posture or faulty breathing patterns can lead to trigger points in the obliques.

Digestive or genitourinary dysfunction is a more common symptom of trigger points in the abdominals than muscular pain. When there are trigger points in all three muscles, heartburn and pain in the upper stomach may be present. Trigger points can be to blame for gas, bloating, and indigestion. Trigger points in internal oblique cause spasm of the urinary sphincter and frequent urination or urine retention. Trigger points can also cause groin pain and pain in the testicles in men as well as menstrual cramps in women.

It's important to see your physician if you are having any of these symptoms. However, it's also important to remember that if medical tests show that your organ function is normal and if your symptoms don't respond to medical treatment, feel for muscular trigger points in the abdominals. Work on them, release them, and see how you respond.

It's difficult to distinguish the obliques and transversus from one another when you are feeling for trigger points. Lie on your back with your head on a low pillow. Starting at the lower border of your ribs, massage the sides of your abdomen down toward the crest of the pelvis and your groin. Feel for areas of muscle that are sore and taut and feel like tight bands. Feel for tender spots within those bands. Take your time and try to examine the abdominals throughout your torso, searching for those taut bands. When you find them, press with your fingers to release them. If you inhale while you are pressing the band, the outward pressure of your in-breath will provide some resistance to your pressure. This will help to release the band.

Follow these sessions with stretches. Stretch the obliques and transversus by standing with your back about twelve inches from a wall. Twist your upper body and place the palms of your hands on the wall. Hold the position for a count of fifteen to twenty. Repeat the stretch, this time twisting your body to the opposite side.

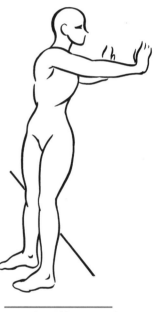

Stretch: Obliques and Transversus abdominis

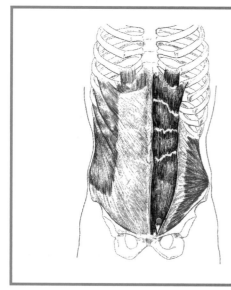

The Abdominals

Rectus Abdominis

Rectus abdominis and trigger points

RECTUS ABDOMINIS attaches from the lower end of the breastbone and the adjacent ribs to the pubic bone. A well-developed rectus creates the "six-pack" look.

Rectus bends the torso forward; trigger points can develop from overuse or strain. The scarring that results from abdominal surgery can also lead to trigger points in rectus. Trigger points may also develop in response to the presence of disease or dysfunction of any abdominal organ. If pain is accompanied by appetite, digestion, or elimination problems, it's best to check in with your doctor.

When trigger points are present in the upper sections of rectus, you might experience pain across the middle of your back; trigger points in the lower sections of rectus can produce pain across the lower part of your back. Pain may also be experienced in the lower abdomen, on the same side as the trigger points. In addition to pain, digestive symptoms such as heartburn, bloating, gas, nausea, and lower abdominal cramping are quite common. Menstrual cramps are also associated with trigger points in rectus.

To locate trigger points and taut bands in rectus, lie on your back with your head on a thin pillow. Massage across the vertical bands of muscle on both sides of the midline of your body, starting just below your breastbone and moving down toward your pubic bone. Feel for taut bands with tender spots. Press into a taut band; breathe slowly and allow the outward movement of the musculature to provide a gentle resistance to your compressions.

Follow your work with stretching. Lie on the floor on your belly with your palms down at the level of your chest. Raise your upper body,

Stretch: Rectus abdominis

Torso Pain

supporting its weight with your arms. Arch your head and neck toward the ceiling, keeping the hips, legs, and feet relaxed on the floor. Hold this position for a count of fifteen to twenty. Release the stretch by bending the elbows and slowly bringing the upper body down.

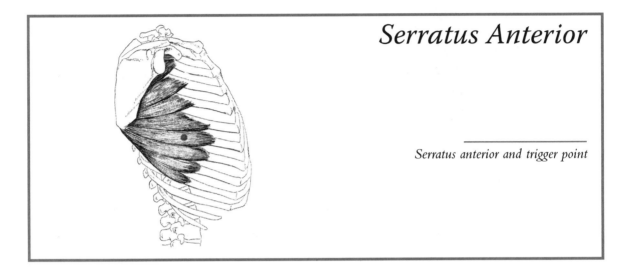

Serratus Anterior

Serratus anterior and trigger point

SERRATUS ANTERIOR connects the shoulder blade to the rib cage, attaching to the inner border of the shoulder blade and to the side of the rib cage on the first eight or nine ribs. Serratus anterior resembles little fingers of muscle that interconnect with the fibers of external oblique on the side of the rib cage. When serratus anterior contracts it pulls the shoulder blade forward across the rib cage. It also works to stabilize the shoulder blade in pushing actions such as push-ups. People whose shoulder blades "wing out" off the rib cage have weak serratus anteriors.

Running too much or too fast will strain serratus anterior and lead to trigger points; one of the symptoms associated with trigger points in serratus is the "stitch in the side" that occurs sometimes when you take a deep breath while running. Serratus anterior is also strained during push-ups or chin-ups or heavy overhead lifting. Bodybuilders who are pushing heavy weight while striving for increased bulk are at risk for developing trigger points in serratus. Severe coughing may also lead to serratus trigger points.

When trigger points are present in this muscle, pain will be experienced on the side of the rib cage and between the spine and the shoulder blade, near the lower edge of the blade. Pain may radiate down the inside of the arm all the way to the pinky and ring fingers. Pain can be intense and persistent but will generally be unaffected by movement. Shortness of breath—the feeling that you can't take a

Torso Pain

■

deep breath without pain because you can't expand your chest—is a symptom associated with trigger points in serratus anterior.

Trigger points can develop in any one of the slips of serratus anterior, so you'll have to palpate this muscle thoroughly. Lie on your pain-free side with your head supported by a pillow. Rest your upper arm over your head. Place your fingertips of your other hand in the armpit of the side to be palpated. The palm of your hand is flat against the side of your rib cage. Palpate the upper slips of serratus anterior with your fingertips and then slowly move your hand down, rib by rib, palpating slips of muscle and feeling for taut bands and tenderness. The most common trigger point is found on the same level as your nipple, but check the muscle as completely as you can in order to make sure that you identify all the trigger points.

You'll be able to release the trigger points using fingertip pressure. You won't have to press too hard, because the muscle is not very thick. Breathe through the soreness and wait for a gentle release. Repeat this process a couple of times a day until you no longer feel tender spots in the muscle.

To stretch serratus after you've worked on it, sit on a chair and place the arm of your painful side over the back of the chair, holding on to the seat of the chair with your other hand to support you. Slowly turn your torso away from the arm that's over the back of the chair. Hold this position for a good count of twenty and then release.

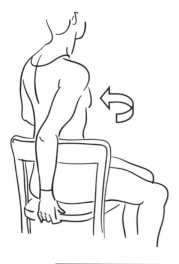

Stretch: Serratus anterior

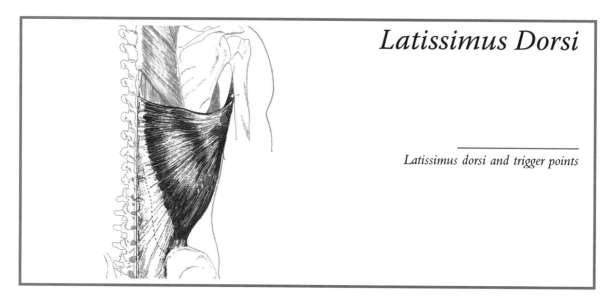

Latissimus Dorsi

Latissimus dorsi and trigger points

LATISSIMUS DORSI is a broad, thin muscle that covers the lower and mid back before it thickens at the level of the armpit. As pectoralis major forms the front wall of the armpit, latissimus dorsi forms its back wall. Latissimus dorsi works to bring the arm down and in toward the chest and extend it behind the body line. Think of freestyle swimming. That forward and downward motion is the work of the lats.

Consider the extent to which these muscles are used in athletics—weight lifting, skiing, hiking, gymnastics, swimming, tennis, basketball, pitching, throwing—the motion of bringing the arm down and in toward the chest is involved in so many sport actions. Trigger points can develop as a function of overusing the latissimus in the course of its action or by using it to support a weight with the arms outstretched. Think of the male dancer again; when he carries his partner overhead across the stage he's supporting a weight with his arms outstretched, and working his lats quite hard as he is doing so.

The pain associated with latissimus dorsi trigger points is an annoying ache at the bottom of the shoulder blade and the surrounding mid back area that neither activity nor rest changes. There might also be pain up to the back of the shoulder and down the inside of the arm, possibly to the ring finger and pinky. You may not be able to reach forward and up without pain.

The most common trigger points in latissimus dorsi lie in the muscle mass that forms the back wall of the armpit. Reach under your arm and feel for the sharp outside edge of the shoulder blade. You can use your thumb and fingers to grasp the mass of muscle lying right next to it. The trigger points of latissimus dorsi can be found on the back of that muscle mass. You can massage with your fingers or you can use a small ball to compress the muscle. Lie on the floor and place the ball between your shoulder blade and the floor. Relax and breathe as you allow gravity to drop your body weight into the ball, compressing the trigger point.

To stretch latissimus dorsi, reach both arms overhead. Grasp the wrist of the hand on the painful side with the opposite hand. Pull the wrist and arm away from the painful side, bending the torso to that side. Hold this position for a count of ten to fifteen.

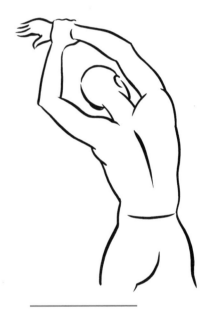

Stretch: Latissimus dorsi

Low Back, Buttock, Hip, and Thigh Pain

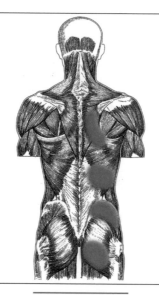

Pain pattern: Erector spinae

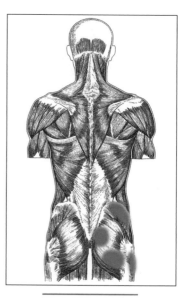

Pain pattern: Quadratus lumborum

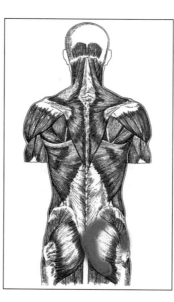

Gluteus maximus

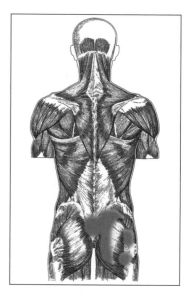

Gluteus medius

Pain pattern: The Gluteals

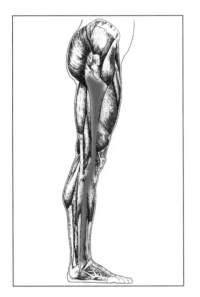

Gluteus minimus

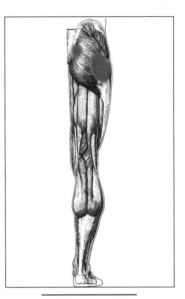

Gluteus minimus

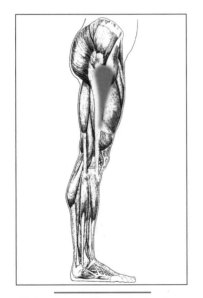

Pain pattern: Piriformis

Pain pattern: The Gluteals

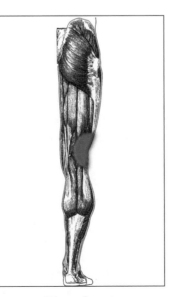

Pain pattern: Tensor fasciae latae

Biceps femoris

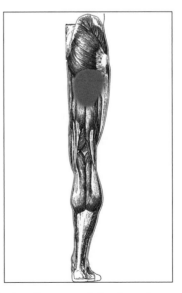

Semitendinosus and Semimembranosus

Pain pattern: Hamstrings

Low back, buttock, hip, and leg pain: something that a majority of adults has unfortunately experienced. And once experienced, it isn't forgotten. Back pain is a major cause of loss of activity for adults; it is as common as the common cold. The muscles addressed in this section are involved in almost every activity you can think of, and yet are most often overlooked as the source of sciatic pain, a term that describes the location of pain in the buttock, thigh, and / or leg. The numerous muscles that lie in the area of the lumbar spine or low back and that form the muscle mass of the buttocks and hips are more frequently involved in pain in this region than is generally assumed. These muscles are involved in much of the heavy work we do: bending, lifting, digging, vacuuming. They are overburdened by awkward positions—twisting to one side to lift an object off the floor, for example. They are overworked by standing too long, sitting too long, carrying a burden that is just too heavy, and carrying an emotional burden that is heavy as well. The muscles in this region are stressed by poor posture while standing or sitting and the effects on posture as we age.

For those of us who are athletes and dancers, the low back and the hip are a source of power and force. The stability provided by the back muscles and the force provided by the muscles of the buttock and hip supply the power, speed, and precision that create optimal performance. We want to play, we want to move, and we want to get stronger and better at our sport. Unfortunately, it is often during these efforts that overuse injuries occur to these muscles: running too hard and too long; practicing too hard and too long; twisting over and over to perfect a golf swing; straining to accomplish something that is just a bit outside of our capability.

Some of us are weekend warriors. We are busy being "productive" all week long, and as a result we sit for too many hours, we don't eat well, and we don't get enough sleep. Many of us aren't in the best physical condition. We believe that we can do far more than we can do—our minds are in our twenties and thirties but our bodies are in their forties and fifties. Our muscles are tight, sore, and weak. Still, when the weekend comes we play a grueling game of softball or several sets of tennis, pushing our bodies to perform as best they can. Overworking an unconditioned muscle this way is a source of injury, one of the most common.

There are other sources of injury that have nothing to do with sports, and we all have those experiences at one time or another too. Overuse can occur from shoveling snow or digging in a garden, or from repeated heavy or awkward lifting. Trauma from falls or automobile accidents can produce injuries to the muscles of the back and hip. And as much as overactivity can be a liability, immobility can take a toll on the muscles too. Immobility can be a source for trigger points. At one time or another we all take long plane rides, spend long hours in front of a computer, or have to spend time on the couch recovering from an injury. Immobility tends to shorten and weaken the muscles of the back and hip.

While occasionally you might be able to identify the specific event that was source of your back pain, some of the time you may not. It's not unusual to hear someone cry "But I didn't *do* anything! I just bent over the sink to brush my teeth and my back went out!" The body was finally reacting to an accumulation of muscular stresses and strains.

The list of sources for pain in this region of the body is quite diverse, encompassing both overexertion and lack of exertion. The remedy is care and conditioning of the muscles throughout our day and throughout our lives, regardless of whether or not we are athletes. Stretching and strengthening is extremely important as we move through our lives. If we want to move comfortably through our older years, we have to move regularly throughout all our years.

Low Back, Buttock, Hip, and Thigh Pain

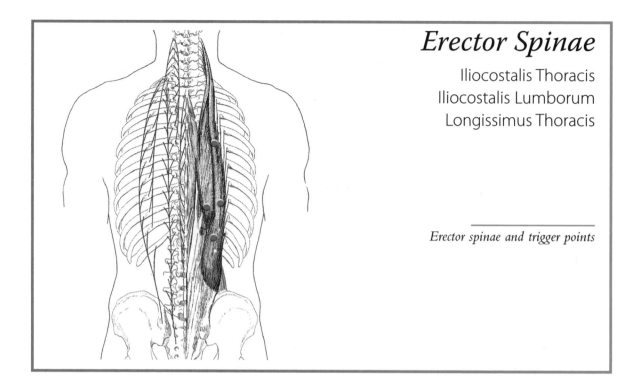

Erector Spinae

Iliocostalis Thoracis
Iliocostalis Lumborum
Longissimus Thoracis

Erector spinae and trigger points

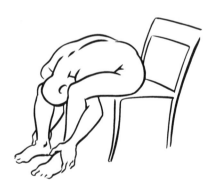

Stretch 1: Erector spinae

Low Back, Buttock, Hip,
and Thigh Pain

■

THE ERECTOR SPINAE GROUP is the most superficial of the paraspinal muscles, muscles that lie on either side of the spine. This group of muscles is considered to be the "true" back muscles. The function of erector spinae is to maintain upright posture and to move and protect the spinal column.

Erector spinae extends from a single broad attachment at the sacrum, the upper part of the pelvis, and each of the five lumbar vertebrae in the low back upward to each of the ribs and the vertebrae adjacent to them, the thoracic vertebrae. When these muscles work bilaterally they straighten the back and extend the spine; when only one side is in action they work with the abdominals to bend the torso to the side.

The most common source of trigger points in erector spinae is from overloading the muscles through straining while lifting improperly. Bending forward from the hips to lift an object from the floor, rather than reaching from bent knees, places a excessive load on these muscles. Straining to have a bowel movement and coughing also produce a strong contraction of erector spinae. The erector spinae is in a continual state of contraction in the person who has a strongly arched low back. This chronic overload may lead to trigger points. Immobility can also lead to trigger points in erector spinae: sitting for extended periods of time without break can cause trigger points to develop. Whether sitting at a desk or on an airplane, it's important to move around at regular intervals to prevent restriction of erector spinae.

Trigger points can develop at just about any level of the muscle. The pain that is produced can be either close to the trigger point or referred farther from the trigger point, along the course of the muscle. Trigger points in the low back portion of erector spinae tend to refer pain to the low back and buttocks; trigger points in the rib cage portion of the muscle tend to refer pain upward, higher in the back. Some trigger points even produce pain in both the back and the front of the torso. Pain is frequently accompanied by restricted motion. Both forward bending and sidebending may be uncomfortable. If trigger points are present in both sides of erector spinae at the level of your lowest rib, you might not be able to get out of a chair or climb stairs comfortably.

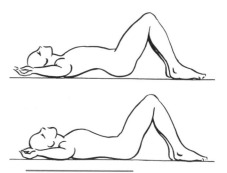

Stretch 2: Erector spinae

The easiest way to treat your own trigger points is to lie on a tennis ball. You can make a convenient treatment device by placing two tennis balls in a sock and tying the sock so the balls stay together. Lie on the floor and place the balls, one on each side of the spine, at the level of the trigger point. Relax and just let gravity do its work. Breathing deeply helps to relax the muscle. Each time you exhale, allow your body to drop down further onto the balls. Stay at one point for several minutes and then move the balls to another level of the spine. It may take some time but the muscle will slowly relax.

Follow up with stretches. Do any one that you can manage, and then work up to the other two.

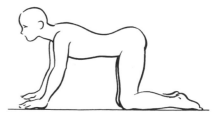

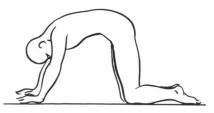

Stretch 3: Erector spinae

1. Sit comfortably on a chair with your feet placed flat on the floor. Fold your torso toward the floor, reaching forward and down with your arms. A key here is to allow your head and neck to drop down and hang loosely. Hold this position for a count of twenty to thirty. Slowly lift back up to a seated position.

2. Lie on your back. Bend your knees and place the soles of your feet on the floor. Exhale and slowly drop your low back toward the floor. Hold for a count of five and then release. Repeat this several times, making sure that you aren't pulling your belly in and tucking your pelvis.

3. Position your body on your hands and knees. Arch your back, lifting both your head and your buttocks toward the ceiling. Hold this position for a count of five. Then round your back, aiming your head and your tailbone for the floor. Hold again for a count of five. Alternate these two movements three or four times.

Low Back, Buttock, Hip, and Thigh Pain

Following treatment and stretches, use a moist heating pad or take a hot bath to hydrate the muscle. It will help enormously! If you're using a moist heating pad, lie on your belly and place a pillow underneath your ankles. This will put a bend in your knees and help to take pressure off the low back.

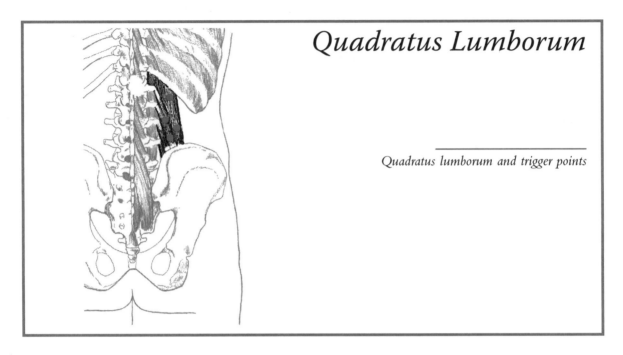

Quadratus Lumborum

Quadratus lumborum and trigger points

QUADRATUS LUMBORUM is one of the muscles that is most commonly involved in low back pain; in fact it is the most frequent muscular source of low back pain. This small, deep muscle lies in the small of the back. Its upper attachments are to the tiny, floating twelfth rib at the very bottom of the rib cage and to the sides of the first four lumbar vertebrae. Its lower attachment is to the top of the pelvis, the iliac crest.

Quadratus lumborum gives your lumbar spine stability while you are standing. When it contracts it bends the lumbar spine to the side and it hikes the hip upward. It's active during breathing, keeping your rib cage down while you inhale. It's especially active during a forced exhalation or when you cough or sneeze.

Overloading the muscle is often the source of trigger points in quadratus lumborum. Bending to one side and lifting something at the same time is a common instigator, as is simply bending and twisting at the same time. Lifting something heavy in an awkward position can overload quadratus. Quadratus trigger points are extremely common following the trauma of an automobile accident. Jogging or walking on a slanted surface such as a crowned road or a beach, where one side is higher than the other, can lead to restriction in quadratus on the side of the body that is walking on the high side of the road. Because the slant tilts the hips, quadratus will contract more on one side than the other. The same situation takes place in a woman's body when she uses one arm to cook while supporting her toddler on her opposite hip. (How many mothers have done that, myself included!) And the game of golf, with its repeated bending, twisting, and forceful rotation to the opposite side, is a classic recipe for quadratus trigger points.

When trigger points are present in quadratus, pain will be felt in the pelvis. One group of trigger points produces pain in the iliac crest and the hip; another produces pain on the side of the sacrum and deep within the center of the buttock. Pain might also be felt in the groin.

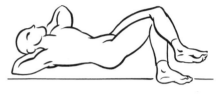

Stretch 1: Quadratus lumborum

When trigger points are present in quadratus the pain can be deep, aching, and unrelenting. Pain is worse when standing. You may need to support your body's weight with your arms in order to turn over in bed or to get out of a bed or a chair or to stand. You may not be able to bend forward without pain. If pain is very severe, you can give yourself a bit of relief, enough to help you stand or walk, by pressing the top of your pelvis while you are standing. Press in and then down with your hands and arms.

If there are trigger points in quadratus you might notice that, in addition to pain, one leg is shorter than the other. Quadratus is a "hip hiker"; it pulls the hip up. When the muscle is shortened and has trigger points, that pull will produce what appears to be a short leg. Once the muscle is released the leg-length discrepancy will disappear.

The quadratus lies within the soft tissues between your last rib and the top of your pelvis. It can be massaged while standing but it is most clearly identified lying down. Lie on your pain-free side with a thin pillow underneath your head and another beneath your waist, between the top of your pelvis and your ribs. Position your legs so that your upper knee is lying behind the back of your lower knee. Feel the soft space between the top of your pelvis and your lower ribs. Use your thumb to identify the top of your pelvis, the iliac crest. Trace the top of your pelvis back toward your spine. It is here that you will find the tender, taut bands of quadratus. Inhale deeply as you are working. This will engage the quadratus, making it easier to identify.

Press in toward your spine to work on the quadratus. From here trace the taut bands up toward the bottom of your rib cage. Press

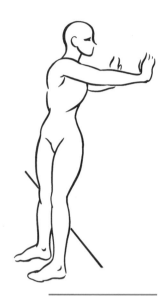

Stretch 2: Quadratus lumborum

directly into the taut bands to release them. Frequent work on the quadratus, two or three times daily for several days, may be needed to completely release the muscle.

Stretching is extremely important for releasing quadratus. Lie on your back with your feet on the floor and your knees bent. Cross the knee of your pain*less* leg over the knee of your pain*ful* leg. Use the upper leg to pull the lower leg away from the painful side. Pulling away from the painful side will stretch the restricted muscles that are causing the pain. If your pain is on the right side, cross your left leg over your right and pull your right leg down toward the left side. Hold this stretch for a slow count of fifteen to twenty. Repeat it several times daily.

You can also stretch quadratus while standing. Stand with your back approximately 12 inches away from a wall. Twist your upper body to place both arms on the wall behind you.

It's very common for trigger points to develop in gluteus medius and minimus (page 117) when there are trigger points in quadratus lumborum. Make sure you check out those muscles for trigger points after you've worked on quadratus.

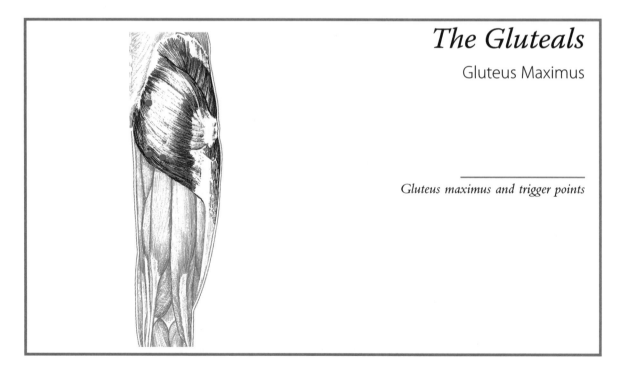

The Gluteals
Gluteus Maximus

Gluteus maximus and trigger points

OF THE THREE GLUTEAL MUSCLES, gluteus maximus is the one that we most often think of when we talk about the "glutes." The evolution of the gluteus muscles allowed for our typically human upright posture. The development of the large, thick, fleshy gluteus maximus allowed us to stand upright, which freed the hands to develop the manual dexterity unique to humans. Gluteus maximus attaches to the pelvis at the back of the iliac crest and to the side of the sacrum and coccyx. It attaches to the femur (the long thigh bone) and the iliotibial band, a broad, thin band of fascia that runs from the top of the thigh to the knee.

Gluteus maximus extends the thigh, an action that is used in activities such as climbing stairs, walking hills, and doing an arabesque, and it laterally rotates the thigh, turning the knee outward. It is most active during strenuous activities such as running, jumping, stair climbing, hill climbing, and rising from a seated position. Contractions of the gluteus maximus function to control certain movements: sitting down, walking down stairs, stooping and bending. An interesting side note: When you are standing or walking the gluteus covers your sitz bones, but when you are sitting upright, as in a straight-backed chair, the muscles slide above the sitz bones so you aren't sitting on your glutes. When you slouch in a chair you are sitting on your glutes.

Trigger points often develop in gluteus maximus from direct impact (a fall) or from muscle overload in trying to prevent a fall. They also develop from walking uphill, particularly in a position in which your body is leaning forward—the posture that hikers typically assume as they ascend a steep slope. Swimming freestyle can contribute to trigger points in gluteus maximus because of the forceful and repeated extension of the legs. The dancer practicing an arabesque or attitude is also at risk for trigger points because of the repeated demands on the muscle. Compressing gluteus maximus while sitting in a slouched position or by keeping a thick wallet in your back pocket will contribute to the development of trigger points as well.

When trigger points are present in gluteus maximus, pain is generally felt in the buttock. A trigger point close to your sacrum will produce pain right at the sacrum and in the portion of your buttock closest to it. A more common trigger point, located just above the sitz bone (the ischial tuberosity), produces generalized buttock pain with tenderness deep within your buttock. Sitting may be so uncomfortable that it will feel as if you are sitting on a hot knife. A trigger point closest to the tailbone (the coccyx) at the bottom of

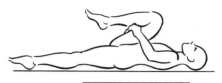

Stretch: Gluteus maximus (knee to homolateral shoulder)

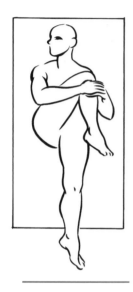

Stretch: Gluteus maximus (knee to opposite shoulder)

the sacrum produces pain right there. If this trigger point is present coccyx pain will be worse when you sit, even though your coccyx is not in contact with the chair at all. Any of these trigger points in gluteus maximus will shorten the muscle and make it very difficult to reach down and touch the floor when you're sitting in a chair.

To identify the trigger points in gluteus maximus you'll first have to locate a couple of bony landmarks: the sacrum and the ischial tuberosities. The sacrum is the flat triangular bone at the base of the spine. The ischial tuberosities are your sitz bones, the bones you sit on (hence the colloquial name). If you place your hands palms up under your buttocks when you are sitting on a chair and then shift your hips back and forth a bit, you will feel the shifting of your hard sitz bones.

Identify gluteus trigger points either standing or lying on your side. Then lie on your back to work on the trigger points. The most common trigger point is generally just above the sitz bones. Feel for the sitz bone and then feel for taut bands of muscle just above it. Once you've found a tender spot, place a small hard ball, such as a squash ball, right on it between your body and the floor. Relax, breathe, and let gravity do its work. The pressure will release the trigger point after a couple of minutes. Next, check out the area beside your sacrum. If there are tender spots in the muscle there, repeat the process with the squash ball. You can do the same thing with the trigger point located in the muscle just beside and below the tailbone, the bottom tip of the sacrum. Just make sure that you place the ball in contact with the muscle, not the coccyx. If a trigger point exists there, you will feel the tenderness and you can release it the same way as the other two.

To stretch gluteus maximus, lie on your back. Grasp the back of the knee of the painful side and pull it up toward the shoulder on the same (homolateral) side. Hold this for a count of fifteen to twenty. Then grasp the top of that knee and draw it toward the opposite shoulder. Hold that position for a count of fifteen to twenty as well. Do both stretches regularly throughout the day to lengthen gluteus maximus.

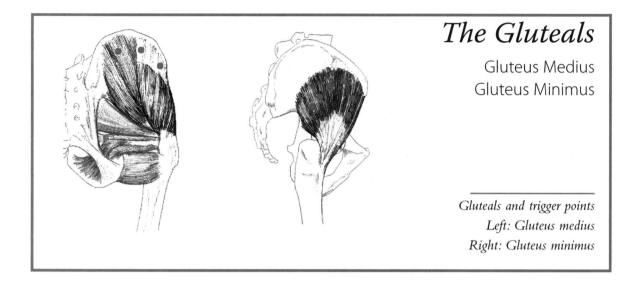

The Gluteals

Gluteus Medius
Gluteus Minimus

Gluteals and trigger points
Left: Gluteus medius
Right: Gluteus minimus

GLUTEUS MEDIUS AND GLUTEUS MINIMUS, the two smaller gluteal muscles, are so closely aligned in terms of location, function, and self-treatment that it makes sense to look at them at the same time. When we think of the gluteal muscles we think of muscles that cover the buttocks; however, these two muscles lie on the side of the pelvis—the hip—one on top of the other.

To locate gluteus medius and gluteus minimus, place the heel of your hand at your hip on the top of the curved brim of the pelvis, with your middle finger in line with what would be your outside pants seam. When your hands are placed this way they are lying over gluteus medius and gluteus minimus. These muscles connect the outside of the pelvis, just underneath its brim, to the greater trochanter, the bony top of the long thigh bone (the femur). With your hands in this position your fingertips fall on the greater trochanter; you can feel its movement as you move your thigh inwardly (internally rotating it) and outwardly (externally rotating it). Gluteus minimus lies just underneath gluteus medius.

Gluteus medius and minimus are powerful abductors of the thigh—they move the thigh, and therefore the leg, away from the body. Their fibers also rotate the thigh both inwardly and outwardly. If you walk around while keeping your hands placed over these two muscles you'll feel them contract, first one side and then the other, as your weight shifts from one leg to the other. The muscles are performing an essential function: stabilizing the pelvis during walking.

Overuse, strain, and injury in sports and dance are major sources of trigger point development in gluteus medius and minimus. Jogging or walking on a soft or sandy surface, running, and vigorous dance

Low Back, Buttock, Hip,
and Thigh Pain

■

117

such as aerobics or African dance can produce an overuse injury. So can ballet and tai chi or other martial arts that require keeping your body weight on one leg for periods of time. Trauma from an impact or fall is also a source of trigger points. Carrying heavy weight on one side can strain the gluteals and lead to trigger points. Lying in the fetal position or sitting for extended periods of time either with your legs crossed or your knees higher than your hips can be problematic for these gluteals as well. It's very common for trigger points to develop in gluteus medius and gluteus minimus when there are trigger points present in quadratus lumborum. If you find trigger points here, feel for trigger points in quadratus lumborum (page 112) as well.

While trigger points in gluteus medius and minimus develop largely in the same way, their pain patterns are somewhat different. When trigger points are present in gluteus medius, pain is experienced across the top of the back of the pelvis and the sacrum. Pain can also be experienced on the outer part of the buttock, occasionally into the upper part of the back of the thigh. You might have pain while walking, when lying on your back or your painful side, or when sitting slouched in a chair.

Like gluteus medius, gluteus minimus trigger points cause pain in the buttock, but there is also pain into the thigh and down the leg. Trigger points in the back portion of the muscle cause pain down the back of the thigh and into the back of the calf. Trigger points in the front portion of the muscle will be experienced on the side of the buttock and down the outside of the thigh and lower leg, possibly as far down as the ankle. Pain from trigger points in gluteus minimus can be excruciating. You may not be able to walk without a limp, you may not be able to get out of a chair, and you may not be able to roll over in bed without pain. Crossing one leg over the other can be very difficult because of restriction in your painful hip.

The location of pain produced by gluteus minimus closely resembles what is known as sciatica. The term *sciatica* is a description of the presence of pain in the area of the buttock, thigh, and leg—sciatica is a symptom, not a diagnosis. Sciatic pain may be due to nerve impingement. Symptoms related to nerve impingement include numbness, tingling, and loss of strength and/or function in the leg and foot. Pain due to the presence of trigger points is deep and aching; there is neither loss of strength nor function in the leg and foot. Diagnostic tests performed by your physician will identify whether your pain is from nerve impingement. If it is not, it is most likely due to trigger points.

Release of trigger points in gluteus medius and minimus can be accomplished with the use of a tennis ball or another kind of small hard ball. First locate the taut bands and trigger points. Lie on your pain-free side with your knees slightly bent. Massage into the hip, the area underneath the brim of the pelvis and down toward the top of the thigh bone, to find taut bands and tender spots. Once you've identified any trigger points, roll onto your painful side to compress them using a tennis ball between your body and the floor. Allow gravity to do its work. Roll onto the front aspect your hip to compress the trigger points in the front portion of these gluteals. You will know when you're in the right place; it will hurt like the dickens. But if you hold the position and breathe and relax for a couple of minutes, the trigger points and soreness will slowly begin to release.

Follow these sessions with stretches. Support your balance by holding on to a wall or table. Cross your painful leg behind the painless leg. Bend the knee of the painless leg as you slide the other away from the torso. Aim your painful hip toward the floor. Hold this position for a count of twenty to thirty. You can stretch these gluteals in the standing position by crossing a pointed foot of your painless leg over the ankle of your painful side. Bend the knee of your painful leg into the back of your painless leg and shift your weight into your painful hip at the same time. If there is restriction in your hip you will feel the stretch between the pelvis and the top of the femur. Hold this position for a count of fifteen to twenty and repeat it several times daily for a complete release.

Trigger points often develop in muscles that lie within the pain pattern produced by other muscles. Gluteus minimus produces a pain pattern that covers the calf. This may result in trigger points in gastrocnemius (page 156) and soleus (page 158). If your pain extends all the way into your calf, make sure to check out these muscles to make sure that trigger points aren't present there as well.

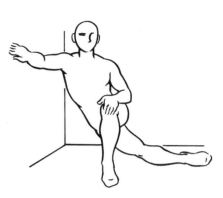

Stretch 1: Gluteus medius and Gluteus minimus

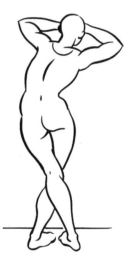

Stretch 2: Gluteus medius and Gluteus minimus

Low Back, Buttock, Hip, and Thigh Pain

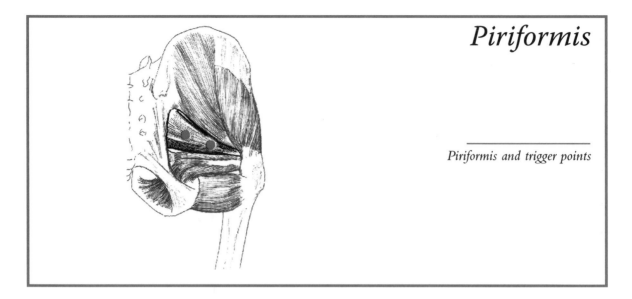

Piriformis

Piriformis and trigger points

PIRIFORMIS lies in the buttock, underneath gluteus maximus. It attaches to the sacrum, the flat bony end of the spinal column, and to the greater trochanter, the bony upper end of the femur (the long thigh bone). Every dancer has heard of the piriformis muscle. It is the muscle that laterally rotates the thigh, producing the turn-out to which dancers aspire. Of all the athletes in every sport or endeavor, only ballet dancers move with their feet pointing toward opposite walls—that is the result of piriformis muscle contraction. Piriformis is highly active during fast walking and running as well as in sports that demand sudden changes in direction: football, tennis, squash, soccer, and basketball. Sports and dance stress piriformis quite a bit.

Trigger points often develop in piriformis in dancers who are trying to maintain the turned-out position of the legs and feet. They are keeping the muscle in contraction for extended periods of time. That lateral rotation of the thigh also occurs in driving for lengthy periods as well as during sexual activity. Runners, joggers, and sprinters are all at risk of developing piriformis trigger points because of the muscle's activity during in running. Trigger points can develop from an overload that might occur when slipping or from catching yourself from falling. And direct impact from a fall may produce trigger points here. Arthritis of the hip, a common problem in the aging athlete and dancer, is a source of trigger points as well. When trigger points are present in piriformis, pain is felt in the area of the sacrum, buttock, and hip joint. It might extend down into the back of the thigh and it may extend up into the low back. Sitting, standing, and walking increase the pain.

Low Back, Buttock, Hip, and Thigh Pain

When piriformis develops taut bands and trigger points, it thickens and shortens. As a result, it may compress the large sciatic nerve that lies very close to it. That compression can bring with it some numbness, tingling, and other sensory disturbances throughout the thigh, lower leg, and foot, a condition known as piriformis syndrome. Consulting a physician will help you to determine if these symptoms are related to the piriformis or to some other source. Generally the presence of taut bands and tenderness in the piriformis muscle indicate that the piriformis is the source of the pain.

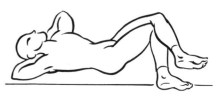

Stretch: Piriformis

To locate piriformis, lie on your side and feel for the edge of your sacrum. Trace an imaginary line between the upper portion of your sacrum and the greater trochanter, the top of the femur. Piriformis lies underneath that line. It is here that you will find taut bands and trigger points in piriformis. The easiest way to release the trigger points is to lie on a tennis ball, placing it just beside the sacrum on the area of tenderness. You will feel the soreness as the weight of your body compresses the tennis ball against your buttock. After a minute or so, move the ball out just a bit in the direction of your hip joint. Lie back, relax, breathe, and let gravity work on that trigger point as well.

Stretch the piriformis after you've worked on it. Lie on your back with your feet on the floor and your knees bent. Cross the knee of your pain*less* side over the knee of your pain*ful* side. Use the upper leg to gently pull the lower leg toward the floor, away from the painful side. Make sure that your hip does not come off the floor. You won't move very much if you're doing this properly, but you will feel a great stretch right across your buttock. Hold this stretch for a count of twenty to thirty. Repeat many times a day for complete release.

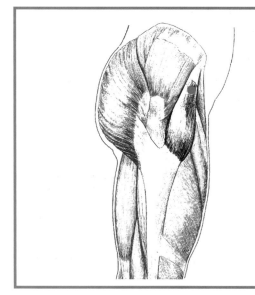

Tensor Fasciae Latae

Tensor fasciae latae and trigger points

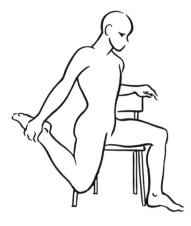

Stretch: Tensor fasciae latae

Low Back, Buttock, Hip, and Thigh Pain

TENSOR FASCIAE LATAE is a small, thick muscle that lies on the side of the pelvis. It attaches to the tibia, the larger of the two lower leg bones, through the long, thin, flat iliotibial band that runs along the outside of your thigh. It acts with other muscles to flex, abduct, and internally rotate the thigh. It helps to stabilize both the pelvis and the knee during walking and running.

Runners and walkers, particularly those who run on sloped or crowned roads, are at risk for developing trigger points in tensor fasciae latae. Jogging, running, or hiking up or down steep slopes may also create trigger points here, particularly if footgear does not provide adequate support. Lying in the fetal position or sitting for long periods of time with your knees higher than your hips can be a source of difficulty for this muscle as well. When trigger points are present in tensor fasciae latae, pain is felt deep in the hip at the area of the greater trochanter, the bony upper end of the long thigh bone. Pain may run down the outside of the thigh toward the knee. You may not be able to sit for long periods of time without pain and walking rapidly may be difficult. Because of tenderness at the greater trochanter, trigger points in this muscle can be easily mistaken for trochanteric bursitis.

To find tensor fasciae latae, lie on your back. Place your hand on the outside of your hip bone. When you press your knees together you should feel the contraction of tensor fasciae latae on the outside of your pelvis. Massage through its fibers to locate taut bands and tender spots. To release them, roll over onto your side and place a small, hard ball between the muscle and the floor. Let the weight of your body compress the trigger points against the ball.

Stretch tensor fasciae latae after you've worked on it. Stand or sit on the edge of a chair. Flex your leg and grasp the ankle with your hand. Rotate your knee outwardly just a bit as you extend your hip and bring your foot up toward your buttock. Hold the stretch for a good count of fifteen to twenty. Repeat this several times a day for a complete release.

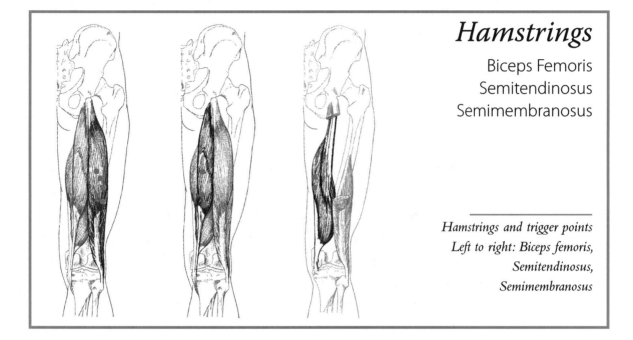

Hamstrings
Biceps Femoris
Semitendinosus
Semimembranosus

Hamstrings and trigger points
Left to right: Biceps femoris,
Semitendinosus,
Semimembranosus

TIGHTNESS OF THE HAMSTRINGS, the muscles that lie on the back of the thigh, is a common source of difficulty for athletes and non-athletes alike. It is the most frequent reason that people are unable to touch their toes in a forward-bending position. Hamstring tightness contributes to the flattening of the normal lumbar curve and to tightness in the muscles of the low back. Hamstring tightness is as common in children as it is in adults.

You can judge for yourself whether your hamstrings are tight. Lie on your back with your legs extended. Lift one leg as high off the floor as you can, keeping both knees straight and your low back on the floor; keep your neck and upper shoulders relaxed. You should be able to aim your toes just about straight up to the ceiling: 80 degrees is "normal."[*] Anything less than that, or if you need to bend your knees or arch your back to bring your leg up, tells you that you've got tight hamstrings.

The hamstring muscles are "two-joint" muscles: they cross the hip

[*]Florence Kendall, Elizabeth McCreary, and Patricia Provance, *Muscles: Testing and Function* (Baltimore: Williams and Wilkins, 1993), 36.

and the knee and therefore act on both. There are three hamstring muscles: biceps femoris, semitendinosus, and semimembranosus. They all attach to the pelvis at the ischial tuberosities, the sitz bones. Biceps femoris attaches below the knee joint to the knobby head of the fibula, the smaller of the two lower leg bones. Semitendinosus and semimembranosus attach below the knee joint, one on top of the other, on the inside of the leg to the back of the tibia, the larger of the two lower leg bones.

The hamstring muscles flex the lower leg (bringing the heel toward the buttock) and extend the thigh, a movement that helps in stair climbing and is essential in keeping the trunk upright. The hamstrings help to prevent you from falling forward while walking.

Compression of the hamstrings often is the source of trigger points. Sitting on a chair or in a car where the seat presses into the back of the thighs is a recipe for hamstring trigger points. Overloading the muscle during sports activities that involve running will produce trigger points: football, basketball, and soccer are such sports. Keeping the hamstrings in the shortened position will produce trigger points—riding an ill-fitted bicycle, practicing poor technique while swimming, taking lengthy hikes or walks down steep hills, and a long period of bed rest all keep the hamstrings in a shortened position for an extended time.

When trigger points are present in biceps femoris, pain will be felt at the back of the outside of the knee; with trigger points in semi-tendinosus and semimembranosus, pain will be felt in the lower part of the buttock and the upper part of the thigh. Pain may extend down into the back of the thigh and the leg as far as the calf. You may have pain while walking, so much so that you might even be limping. Sitting is very uncomfortable; compression of the thighs against the chair seat exacerbates the pain. It's no wonder that hamstring trigger points are often mistaken for sciatica. Because the hamstrings work so closely with the quadriceps, trigger points in the hamstrings will also produce a considerable strain on the quads. This could lead to pain in the front of the thighs and knees. This pain won't be resolved until the tightness in both the hamstrings and the quads is resolved.

You can feel the attachments of the hamstrings while you're sitting down. Their upper attachment is on the ischial tuberosities, the sitz bones. If you place your hands, palms up, under your buttocks when you are sitting on a chair and then shift your hips back and forth a bit you will feel the sitz bones move. To feel the lower attachment of the hamstrings, hold on to your right knee with your right hand around the outside and your left hand around the inside. Place your fingertips into the hollow at the back of your knee. That's the popliteal space. With your hands in this position, your right hand can feel the tendon of biceps femoris and your left hand can feel the tendon of semitendinosus (the tendon of semismembranosus lies beneath semitendinosus, so you won't be able to feel it).

You can work on hamstring trigger points either seated in a chair or sitting on the floor with your leg extended in front of you. Place a small, hard ball such as a tennis ball underneath your thigh at the area of greatest tenderness, most likely in the midpoint of your thigh, either to the left or to the right of center, depending on which of the hamstring is most affected. Let the compression of the muscle work to elongate taut bands of muscle and release the trigger points. Keep at this for a complete release. Treat all the trigger points in the hamstrings for a complete release.

Stretch the hamstrings following treatment. You can stretch the hamstrings sitting on the floor with your leg extended in front of you. You can do this one leg at a time or both legs at the same time. Keeping your knee straight, place the palm of your hand on the bottom of your foot. Pull your toes and your ankle toward you. Hold this position for a good count of fifteen to twenty.

You can also stretch the hamstrings by placing the heel of the leg to be stretched on a step, a ledge, or a chair seat. Make sure that your thigh is directly in front of your hips, not off to the side, and that your toes are pointing straight up. Maintain the angle between your hip and your thigh as you slowly bend forward from the hips. Your leg does not have to be high up to feel the stretch. If the position of your hip and thigh is correct you will feel a great stretch. Hold this for a good count of fifteen to twenty and repeat it regularly throughout the day.

Once you've eliminated your pain through self-treatment and stretching, it's important to work on lengthening the hamstrings to avoid all the pitfalls that shortened hamstrings can bring. You will have to be patient and consistent with the stretching—it may take weeks or months for true lengthening but it is so important that it's worth the time and the effort. Because of the close working relationship between the adductors (page 130) and the hamstrings, it is extremely important to stretch your adductors in addition to your hamstrings to get a complete release. See the adductor stretch on page 131 for instructions.

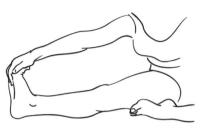

Stretch 1: Hamstrings

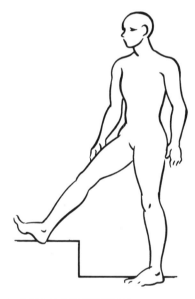

Stretch 2: Hamstrings

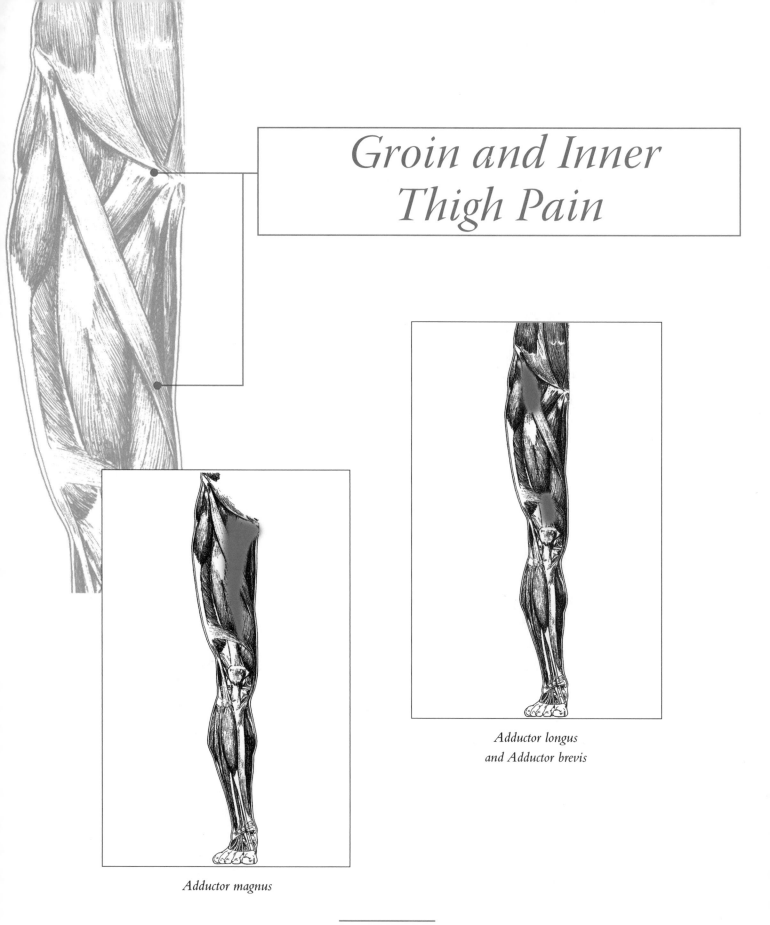

Groin and Inner Thigh Pain

Adductor magnus

Adductor longus
and Adductor brevis

Pain pattern: The Adductors

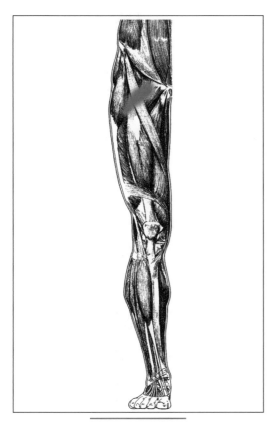

Pain pattern: Pectineus

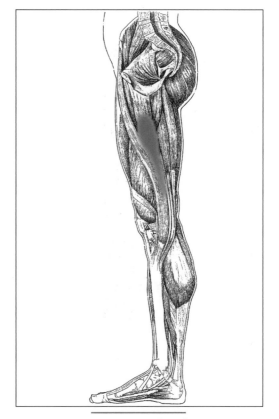

Pain pattern: Gracilis

The word *groin* as it is used here refers to the crease at the junction of the thigh and the trunk. The groin is an area of the body rather than an anatomical structure. It is the area where you can identify the inguinal ligament lying between the pubic bone and the prominent, sharp hip bone on the side of the front of the pelvis. Lying close to the groin are the areas of attachment for many of the muscles that flex the thigh and the trunk and that bring the thigh toward the midline of the body. The primary muscular source of groin and inner thigh pain is injury to the muscles of the inner thigh, the adductors. And it is sadly the case that severe restriction of the muscles of the inner thigh not only lead to inner thigh and groin pain but may lead to deep pelvic pain as well.

Anyone may lose his or her footing on occasion, whether during sports activities, dancing, walking on a snow- or ice-covered sidewalk, or walking down stairs. That misstep can be the source of injury and trigger points in the adductors, as can arthritis of the hip (a huge risk factor for athletes and dancers as we age), sexual activity, or simply staying seated for an extended period of time with the thighs tightly crossed.

Groin and inner thigh pain is a fairly common occurrence in sports endeavors that require quick acceleration and deceleration or side-to-side action. Soccer, hockey, and basketball all fall into this category, as do tennis and other racket sports when they are played vigorously. It is unfortunately the case that many athletes who take part in these sports don't stretch their adductors sufficiently and suffer overload injuries as a result. In athletics and dance we frequently hear that someone has a "pulled groin." The term *pulled groin* actually refers to an overload injury resulting from overstretching, straining, or tearing the inner thigh muscles or the primary hip flexor, the iliopsoas. As with so many other muscular injuries, proper stretching and conditioning of the muscles during training sessions can avert such an injury.

What is generally called a "groin stretch" is actually the combined stretching of the adductors (the inner thigh muscles), the quadriceps

Groin and
Inner Thigh Pain

128

(the muscles of the front of the thigh), and the hamstrings (the muscles of the back of the thigh). The elongation of all of these muscle groups leads to strength and freedom of movement at the hip joint, something to which athletes and dancers alike aspire.

Strength and flexibility in these muscles is highly beneficial to all athletes, dancers, and martial artists. Probably the most common image of flexible inner thigh muscles is the picture of the dancer or gymnast stretching the inner thighs at the barre or on the floor. Flexibility of these muscles is of great value to all athletes, because the greater the flexibility of a muscle the greater its strength. However, for many dancers and martial artists, overstretching and overuse of these muscles can lead to injuries.

Cyclists, rollerbladers, skaters, and skiers are all subject to groin and inner thigh strain due to the parallel thigh position that is required to perform their sports properly. Horseback riders work their inner thighs against resistance (the horse) while riding, much the same way that people using the inner-thigh machine at a gym do. The action that is common to these endeavors results in the overuse of the adductors. This continued action can overload the muscles of the inner thigh and lead to groin pain.

Anyone who has ever worked in circumstances that require squatting for periods of time will attest to the truth that squatting places a great deal of stress on the adductors. At risk are gardeners and carpenters, electricians, and plumbers, who occasionally must work in cramped spaces. Doing squats at the gym to strengthen and develop these muscles can also overuse the adductors.

Overload, overstretch, overuse: these are the main sources of muscle injury to this part of the body.

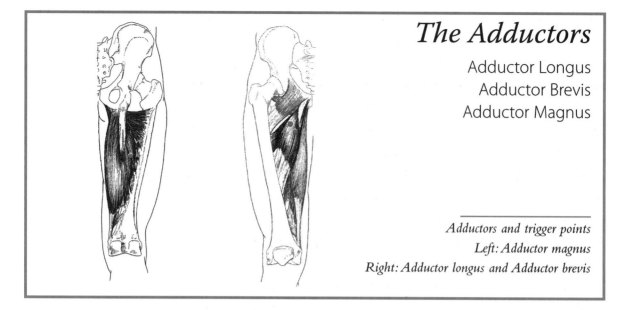

The Adductors

Adductor Longus
Adductor Brevis
Adductor Magnus

Adductors and trigger points
Left: Adductor magnus
Right: Adductor longus and Adductor brevis

THE ADDUCTORS are the inner thigh muscles. They bring the thigh toward the midline of the body. (People often confuse the terms *adductor* and *abductor*. Think of it this way. The muscles on the inside of the thighs, the *add*uctors, add: they bring the legs toward the midline of the body. The muscles on the outer side of the thigh and hip, the *abd*uctors, abduct: they move the legs away from the midline of the body.)

Adductor longus, adductor brevis, and adductor magnus are the muscles that form the bulk of muscle tissue that you feel at the inner thigh. Adductor longus is the most prominent and is the easiest to palpate. Adductor brevis lies beneath adductor longus and cannot be directly palpated.

When trigger points are present in the adductors, groin and inner thigh pain result, and that pain may be accompanied by difficulty abducting your thigh and/or rotating your thigh outwardly. There may be a number of other symptoms as well: deep pelvic pain, rectal or bladder pain, vaginal pain, and possibly pain during sexual intercourse. It is unfortunately the case that a muscular source of these symptoms is often not considered, so people suffer for years while seeking the cause of their pain outside the realm of the muscles.

Adductor longus and adductor brevis connect the pubic bone to the middle section of the long thigh bone, the femur, on the inside of the thigh. Adductor magnus lies behind adductor longus and brevis and connects your sitz bone, the ischial tuberosity of the pelvis, to the back of the femur.

Trigger points in adductor longus and brevis produce pain in the groin and the upper part of the inner thigh. The trigger points in the upper part of adductor longus may even cause stiffness in the knee as well as pain in the inner thigh. Pain is usually experienced while you are active rather than when you are at rest, and pain is worse while standing and bearing weight. Adductor magnus trigger points cause groin pain and inner thigh pain that might extend as far down as the knee. And adductor magnus can be the source of severe, deep pelvic pain that might also include pain at the pubic bone, the vagina, the rectum, and possibly the bladder. Pain from adductor magnus trigger points may be so severe that it can even be mistaken for pelvic inflammatory disease or other diseases relating to the reproductive organs or bladder.

To locate and work on the adductors you'll first have to become familiar with the femoral triangle, a body landmark in the upper thigh. Sit on the floor with your legs extended in front of you. Bend one knee and bring the sole of the foot of that leg to face the inner knee of the extended leg. If this position is not comfortable for you, you can sit on a couch and do the same thing. Your bent leg will rest on the seat of the couch while your other leg will remain in a normal seated position.

Palpate the inner thigh of the bent leg. First find the crease between your thigh and your pelvis. Just at the crease is the inguinal ligament. It goes from the outer edge of your pubic bone up to your hip bone. This ligament forms the base of the femoral triangle. The outer side of the femoral triangle is formed by the sartorius muscle (page 145) and the inner side of the triangle is formed by adductor longus. The floor of the triangle is formed by the lower fibers of iliopsoas (see pages 97 and 140) on the inner side and pectineus on the outer side. The pulse of the femoral artery can be felt in this triangle, as can swollen lymph nodes, nodes that become enlarged when the immune system is fighting off an infection.

Once you've identified adductor longus, grasp it between your thumb and your fingers and palpate it along the inner thigh from the groin to just above the midpoint of the inner thigh. Identify taut bands and trigger points as you palpate; when you locate a trigger point, use your fingers to compress the band and release the trigger point. If your fingers can't quite do the job, a tennis ball or another small, firm ball or one of the many devices on the market today can be used to work on the trigger points. Repetition is key. Keep at it in order to release the muscles completely. You may have to work on the muscle several times a day over the course of days in order to obtain complete release.

To find adductor magnus trigger points, sit in the position described above, but this time move your foot about 10 inches away from your extended leg. Feel for adductor magnus trigger points just behind adductor longus. The bulk of muscle running from the groin throughout the length of the thigh is adductor magnus. Palpate for taut bands and trigger points. Once you've identified them, the easiest way to release them is by sitting on the floor with your legs extended in front of you. Place a tennis ball at the tender area and allow gravity to do its work. Just relax your thigh and leg and compress the muscle against the tennis ball. Repeat this frequently to completely release the muscle.

It's essential to follow up your trigger point release work with stretches. To stretch the adductors, lie with your buttocks against a wall and your legs extended up onto it. Slowly separate your legs to stretch the inner thighs. Hold this position for 30 to 60 seconds and allow gravity to help stretch out your inner thighs. Because of the close working relationship of adductor magnus and biceps femoris (one of the muscles in the hamstrings group), it's extremely important to stretch your hamstrings in addition to your adductors to get a complete release. See the hamstring stretch on pages 125 and 150 for directions.

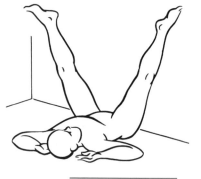

Stretch: Adductors

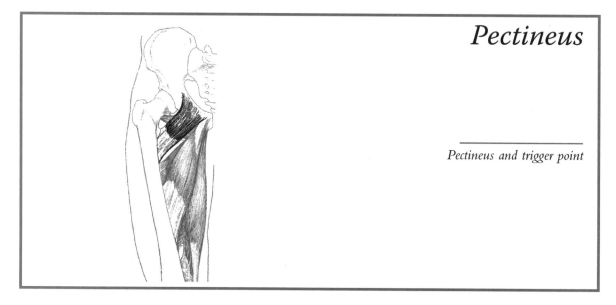

Pectineus

Pectineus and trigger point

PECTINEUS is a small muscle that lies on the upper part of the inner thigh. It connects the pubic bone to the upper thigh. It works with other muscles to adduct the thigh and to flex the thigh at the hip. Trigger points in pectineus produce a deep, persistent, localized pain directly at the groin, just below the inguinal ligament; that pain may extend slightly over the upper part of the inner thigh. Pain from trigger points in pectineus may not become apparent until pain from trigger points in the adductors and/or iliopsoas is alleviated.

A sudden overload to pectineus—an unexpected fall or misstep—is one of the main sources of trigger point development. Trigger points here can develop secondary to hip surgery or a fracture of the femur. They may also develop from the chronic overload that might occur when you are sitting with your thighs tightly crossed or in response to resisting the abduction of the thighs. Think about what it feels like to use the inner-and-outer-thigh machine in the gym. It is exactly that action—pushing against weight to abduct your thighs (separate them) and pushing against weight to adduct your thighs (bring them together)—that might lead to trigger point development in pectineus.

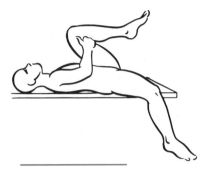

Stretch: Pectineus

To locate pectineus you'll need to find the femoral triangle as described on page 131. Palpate the floor of the triangle. When trigger points are present, pectineus can be identified as a taut band on the inner side of the floor of the triangle. It will feel like a small band of muscle that runs from your pubic bone obliquely toward the middle of your thigh. Find the most tender point in that taut band and then use either direct pressure with your fingers, or even the eraser end of a pencil, to compress the trigger point. Patience and stretch will help you release it. Work on it several times throughout the day and then stretch it by lying on a table or bed and allowing your painful thigh to hang off the side. Bend the thigh of your other leg toward your chest in order to keep your lower spine on the table. Let gravity do its work to stretch the upper groin. Hold this stretch for a count of twenty to thirty and repeat it regularly.

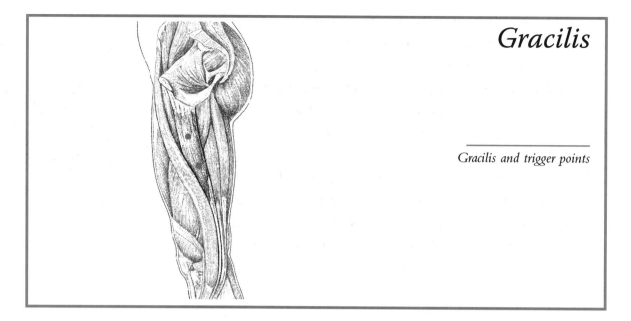

Gracilis

Gracilis and trigger points

GRACILIS is a long, thin strap-like muscle that lies on the inner thigh. It attaches to the pubic bone, runs the length of the inner thigh, and crosses the knee joint to attach to the inner side of the large lower leg bone, the tibia. It works with the adductors to adduct the thigh and it helps to rotate the thigh inwardly when the lower leg is bent.

Gracilis may develop trigger points as a result of a fall or a misstep or when arthritis is present in the hip joint. Trigger points may also develop from overloading gracilis. This might take place while horseback riding, ice skating, doing gymnastics, or when working out in the weight room on the inner-and-outer-thigh machine. Pain is experienced as a hot, stinging superficial pain along the inside of the thigh.

To work on gracilis you'll first have to find its tendon of attachment at the inner knee. Sit on a chair with your body close to a table leg or desk. Your knees are bent and your feet are on the floor. Place your hand at the inside edge of the back of your knee. You'll feel a prominent tendon. That's the tendon of semitendinosus, one of the two hamstring muscles that lie toward the inside of the back of the thigh. Move your hand slightly around toward the inside of your knee and you'll feel another, slightly less prominent, tendon. That's the tendon of gracilis.

Here is where the table leg comes in handy. Press your inner knee against the table leg and gracilis will engage against the resistance. It will then become easy to identify throughout its length and you'll be able to palpate it relatively easily. It will feel like a taut, thin band.

Remain seated but let your thigh relax once you've identified graci-lis. Work along the inner thigh from your knee upwardly toward the groin along the length of gracilis feeling for tender spots within the taut band. When you've located them, press with your fingers, a large pencil eraser, or a small hard ball such as a squash ball to release them. You'll have to repeat this several times in order to obtain complete release.

It's essential to follow up your trigger point release work with stretches. To stretch gracilis, lie with your buttocks against a wall and your legs extended up onto the wall. Slowly separate your legs to stretch the inner thighs. Hold this position for thirty to sixty seconds. Relax, breathe, and allow gravity to help do the work.

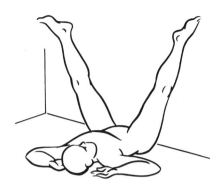

Stretch: Gracilis

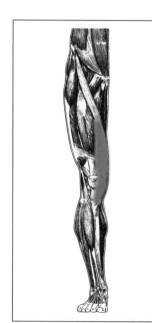

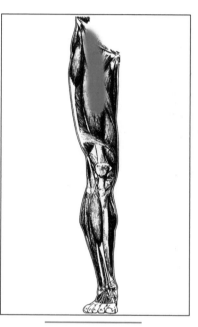

Pain pattern: Iliopsoas

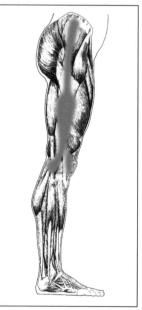

Vastus medialis

Vastus lateralis

Vastus intermedius

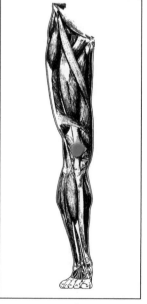

Rectus femoris

Pain pattern: Quadriceps femoris

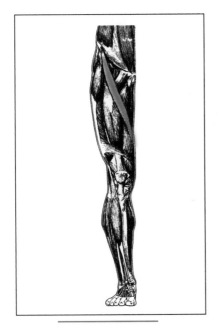

Pain pattern: Sartorius

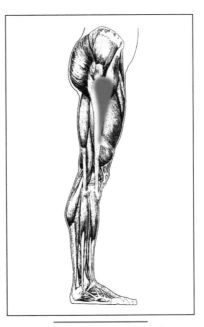

Pain pattern: Tensor fasciae latae

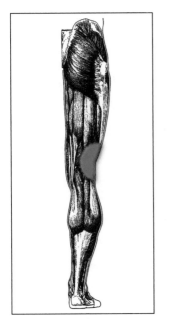

Biceps femoris

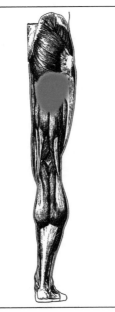

**Semitendinosus
and Semimembranosus**

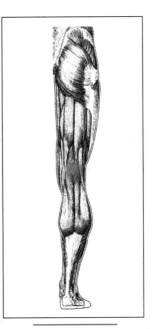

Pain pattern: Popliteus

Pain pattern: Hamstrings

Some of the body's largest and most powerful muscles are the muscles that, when injured, produce thigh and knee pain: the iliopsoas, the body's primary hip flexor; quadriceps femoris, the large extensor of the knee; and the hamstrings, the flexors of the knee. Together these muscles exert the force that move the longest, heaviest, and strongest bone in the body, the femur. The knee joint connects the femur to the two bones of the lower leg: the large tibia, or shin bone, and the smaller fibula lying beside it. The patella, or kneecap, lies just in front of the knee joint. The patella is a small sesamoid bone that develops within the tendon of quadriceps femoris. Its purpose is to protect the tendon from excessive wear and tear and to provide a mechanical advantage to the function of the knee.

Overexertion, overuse, trauma, and poor conditioning are the fundamental reasons for muscular injuries that produce thigh and knee pain. And it is in athletics, dance, martial arts, gymnastics, skiing, climbing, hiking, biking, and track and field that these very powerful muscles are called upon to work their hardest. The combination of demanding endeavors and enthusiastic participants is the recipe for overuse and overexertion.

Seasonal endeavors such as skiing, climbing, and hiking impact these muscles particularly in the early days of a new season. So many of us have had this experience at one time or another in our lives. The skier who gets out there the first weekend with fresh snow can stress these thigh muscles to the point where he or she may not be able to walk well the following day. The annual hiker or gardener may well have the same experience, as does the "weekend warrior." Care needs to be taken to exercise moderately throughout the year or to begin seasonal activities gradually. When the stresses of physical activity meet taut, restricted muscles, injury is bound to occur.

Trauma can occur at any time to anyone. A fall down the stairs or a slip on the ice can lead to the misstep that results in an unexpected pull at the hip or an unfortunate twist of the knee. What is often not considered is that the muscles that work on that joint are affected; trigger points can result. An unexpected twist of the knee will affect the quadriceps, hamstrings, and adductors. Knee pain or dysfunction may result, and yet it may not be recognized as pain that has a muscular source.

Poor muscular conditioning can also be a problem. In the poorly conditioned body the hamstring muscles will tend toward tightness. Tightness of the hamstring muscles is the most common reason for the inability to stretch sufficiently to place the hands on or near the floor in a standing position. Tightness in the hamstrings will overstress the quadriceps, which may ultimately lead to a muscular imbalance that may eventually affect the functioning of the knee. Tight hamstrings can also lead to a flattening of the normal lower back curve and contribute to lower back dysfunction and pain. Hamstring tightness may begin as early as our teen years and continue on throughout our lives, causing increasing dysfunction as we age. Encouraging the habit of exercise that conditions, stretches, and strengthens provides the gift of freedom of movement that may last well into the older years.

The generally sedentary lifestyle that many people have contributes to this tightness. The demands of our day-to-day lives—driving, sitting at a desk, or lengthy air travel—serve to compound the problem. When we sit the iliopsoas is in a state of contraction and the hamstrings are compressed by the chair. Both are sources of trigger points. If your lifestyle requires a great deal of sitting it behooves you to consider ways in which you can interrupt your daily routine to add some movement.

Look at what you do and how you do it. Consider your general level of lower body flexibility and the ease with which you move. Think about your activities and you will figure out how your actions are affecting your muscles.

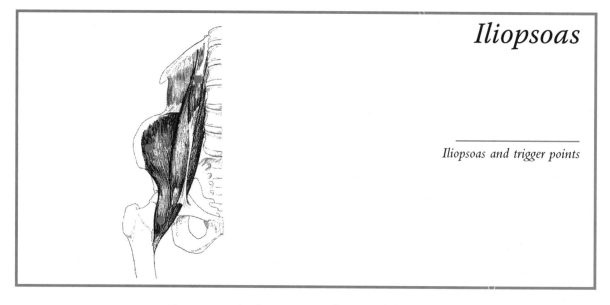

Iliopsoas

Iliopsoas and trigger points

ILIOPSOAS is the primary flexor of the trunk and the most powerful of the thigh flexors. Iliopsoas, often referred to simply as "the psoas," is comprised of two and sometimes three muscles: the psoas, which lies beside the lumbar vertebrae; the iliacus, which lines the inner part of the crests of the pelvis; and psoas minor, which lies in front of psoas major. (Psoas minor is absent in approximately 40 percent of the population.)

Iliopsoas lies on the inside front part of the spine, behind the abdominal organs. It attaches to the sides of the lumbar vertebrae in the low back and to the inside of the pelvis. It passes underneath the inguinal ligament in the groin and attaches to the upper part of the femur, the long bone of the thigh. When the legs are fixed, the contraction of iliopsoas results in bending forward at the hips (flexion of the trunk); when the legs are free, its contraction results in bringing the knee toward the chest (flexion of the thigh on the hip).

Iliopsoas functions in maintaining our upright posture. It works continuously during walking and is considerably active during jogging, running, and kicking. It is highly active during the last 60 degrees of a sit-up. Like the other muscles of the torso, its significance in athletics and dance cannot be emphasized enough.

Trigger points develop in iliopsoas through overload. A repetitive overload would be the repeated forceful flexion of the hip that takes place in dance, gymnastics, jogging, running, hurdling, and sports that involve high kicks—such as those performed by football field kickers. Doing an excessive numbers of sit-ups could also result in trigger points in this muscle for the same reason. A sustained overload would

Thigh and Knee Pain

be sitting for extended periods of time with your knees higher than your hips or lying in the fetal position for extended periods without moving.

When trigger points are present in the upper part of iliopsoas, pain is referred in a vertical pattern alongside the vertebrae of the low back. The pain will be on one side only, the side of the affected muscle. Pain will be much worse while you're standing and will be alleviated when you lie down with your hips and knees bent. When there are trigger points in the lower parts of iliopsoas, pain will be felt in the groin and the front of the upper thigh. A severely restricted iliopsoas will prevent you from standing upright.

Palpating iliopsoas is difficult but not impossible. To find the upper part of iliopsoas, lie on your back. Bend your knees and place your feet on the floor. Shift both knees to the side, *away* from your pain. By lying this way you'll be able to reach beneath some of the abdominal contents to work on iliopsoas. Place your hands at the level of your navel and then shift them a couple of inches to the side, to the outer border of the rectus abdominis (page 102). Press straight down and in toward the midline of your body to palpate taut bands of iliopsoas. Taut bands might feel sore and ropelike. Press deeply along the length of the band from the area just underneath your navel to the inguinal ligament.

Lie on your back with your knees up to palpate trigger points along the inside of the rim of the pelvis. This time you won't have to drop your knees to the side. Find your inguinal ligament (page 131) at your groin. Trace the inguinal ligament upward toward its attachment on the pelvis, your hip bone. Cup your fingers around the bone, trying as best you can to press straight down and then into the inside rim with your fingertips. You'll find trigger points there that refer pain into your groin. You can also release iliopsoas trigger points by applying direct pressure to the portion of the inguinal ligament that is closest to the hip bone.

To find the trigger point that refers pain into the front of your thigh, you'll need to locate the femoral triangle (page 131). Iliopsoas taut bands can be palpated on the outer side of the floor of the femoral triangle. Press gently into the area to release the trigger point. Remember that there are many delicate structures within that triangle, so be sure to exercise care when you compress that region.

As with all muscles, stretching is necessary to obtain complete release. Lie on the edge of a bed or table and let the leg of your

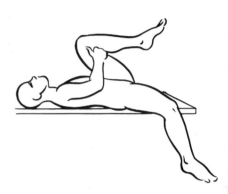

Stretch 1: Iliopsoas

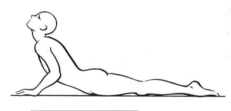

Stretch 2: Iliopsoas

painful side hang off the end. Flex the thigh and leg of your other side to keep your pelvis flat on the table. Let gravity work to stretch the leg down toward the floor. Hold this position for a count of twenty to thirty.

You can also stretch iliopsoas by lying on the floor on your abdomen. Place your hands, palms down, next to your chest. Raise your upper body, supporting it by keeping your weight on your arms. Arch your head and neck toward the ceiling; keep your hips, legs, and feet relaxed on the floor. Hold the stretch for a count of twenty to thirty. Release the stretch by relaxing your arms and bending your elbows to slowly bring your body down to the starting position.

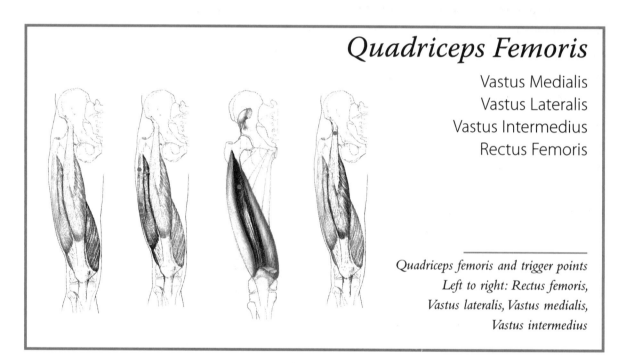

Quadriceps Femoris

Vastus Medialis
Vastus Lateralis
Vastus Intermedius
Rectus Femoris

Quadriceps femoris and trigger points
Left to right: Rectus femoris,
Vastus lateralis, Vastus medialis,
Vastus intermedius

QUADRICEPS FEMORIS is the heaviest, largest, and most powerful muscle in the body. It weighs approximately 50 percent more than the next largest muscle, gluteus maximus. Quadriceps femoris is the primary extensor of the lower leg; the quads straighten the knee. Quadriceps femoris is made up of four separate muscles: vastus medialis, vastus lateralis, vastus intermedius, and rectus femoris. Vastus medialis lies on the inside of the thigh. Vastus lateralis wraps around the outside of the thigh. Vastus intermedius lies against the front of the shaft of the femur. Rectus femoris lies above vastus intermedius along the length of the center of the thigh.

The four quads join together into a thick tendon to attach to the tibia, the larger of the two lower leg bones, just underneath the knee joint. Your kneecap sits just inside that tendon. Of the four muscles that make up quadriceps femoris, only rectus femoris is a two-joint muscle; rectus femoris crosses the hip joint as well as the knee joint. Its upper attachment is to the bony prominence in the front of the pelvis, the hip bone. So in addition to straightening the knee, rectus femoris flexes the thigh; it brings the knee up toward the chest or, when you're standing, its action will bend your hip forward over your thigh.

Trigger points in the quads often occur as a function of injuries, falls, or missteps that twist the knee or as the result of direct trauma to the muscle. Overexertion can produce trigger points—too many squats, deep knee bends, hard and forceful kicks, repeated jumps, running too hard and too fast. Strenuous activities that place a huge demand on your legs can strain the quads and be the source of trigger points: think of dancing, skiing, football, basketball, soccer, running, jogging, hiking, climbing, strenuous cycling, or spin classes. Any activity that requires repeated bending and straightening from the knees or long periods of kneeling can be a problem: gardening, a rigorous game of tennis, or playing the position of catcher in baseball. Because of their close working relationship, tightness in the hamstrings (pages 123 and 148) exacerbates restriction of the quads and makes their release more difficult. The quads won't really let go until the hamstrings are lengthened.

Trigger points in the quads are the most common muscular source of knee pain. They are often overlooked and frequently misdiagnosed. Each of the quads has a different pain pattern and effect on the knee. Trigger points in vastus medialis produce pain in the front and inside of the knee and lower thigh. Sometimes pain will last for days or weeks and then disappear. It's at that point that the knee begins to feel weak and to buckle for no apparent reason. Vastus lateralis can contain many trigger points along the outside of the thigh. Pain may extend the full length of the side of the thigh from the hip to the knee, at the outside of the knee, and toward the back of the knee. You may have difficulty lying on your side at night. The restriction in vastus lateralis also reduces the motion of the kneecap, which can lead to pain and difficulty with walking. Your knee might even lock in a straightened position.

Trigger points in the deepest quad, vastus intermedius, are not as common as trigger points in the others. They usually develop when trigger points have been present in the other quads for some time. When they are present they cause pain that spreads over the front of the thigh. You might have difficulty walking up stairs and straightening your knee after sitting for a period of time. When trigger points are present in rectus femoris pain is experienced in the front of the knee, at the kneecap, and possibly deep in the knee joint. Pain might be severe, deep, and aching, it might extend up over the lower part of the thigh, and it may be worse at night. Walking down stairs can be very difficult if there are trigger points here.

Due to the front-of-the-body location of the quadriceps, treating most of the quad trigger points is fairly straightforward. Rectus femoris trigger points are located high up in the muscle, near its attachment at the hip. To find rectus femoris, sit in a chair and feel for the prominent hip bone in the front of your pelvis just above the crease between your thigh and your torso. Move your fingers slightly below the hip bone and you'll feel thick tendinous tissue. You'll feel this best if you flex your thigh off the chair a bit. What you're feeling here is actually two tendons: the one on the inside is sartorius; the one on the outside is rectus femoris, the one you're looking for. As you flex your thigh you'll feel the separation of the two tendons. Rectus femoris tendon is on the outside.

Follow the tendon down toward your thigh just a bit. Here you'll feel the tendon change to muscle. As you palpate into the muscle you'll begin to feel the taut bands and tenderness of trigger points. It's here that you'll apply pressure. You can use either finger pressure, a small hard ball, or another treatment device to compress the trigger points of rectus femoris. You can work on it in the seated position or you can work on it standing. Whichever position you choose, work on rectus femoris frequently throughout the day to completely release it.

Vastus medialis trigger points are close to the knee on the inside of your thigh. Use your thumb to locate taut bands in the bulk of muscle on the inside of your thigh nearest your knee. You'll find trigger points close to the inside of your knee and up toward the middle of your thigh. Once you've found the taut bands, isolate the trigger points using directed pressure right into them. Your thumb or your fingers work well. Trigger points in vastus lateralis lie throughout the muscle. Trigger points can develop close to the knee, in the midpoint of the thigh, and up by the hip. Massage the outside of your thigh from your hip to your knee to identify taut bands and trigger points.

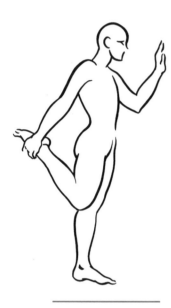

Stretch: Quadriceps

Thigh and Knee Pain

Once you've located areas of tenderness, lie on your side on the floor and place a ball between your thigh and the floor. Gravity will compress the trigger points. You can place the ball in each of the areas where you feel tenderness—there may be quite a few! Take your time and be patient. You'll have to repeat this frequently for a complete release. Vastus intermedius trigger points are hardest to locate because you have to go through rectus femoris to find them. Palpate deeply into your upper thigh to locate these trigger points. Use a small hard ball or another treatment device to compress them.

Stretching the quads is extremely important to obtaining a complete release. To stretch the quads, stand or sit on the edge of a chair. Grasp your ankle, bend your knee, and lift your heel toward your buttock. If you're standing it's important to bring the knee of the leg you are stretching in line with your standing knee. For the greatest stretch, tilt your pelvis forward to prevent flexing your hips. If your quad is so tight that you can't hold your ankle, place your foot on a step or a chair behind you and lean back into it to stretch the quad. Hold the stretch position for a count of twenty to thirty. Repeat this several times a day for a complete release.

Stretching your hamstrings (pages 125 and 150) and your adductors (page 131) is essential for a complete release of your quads.

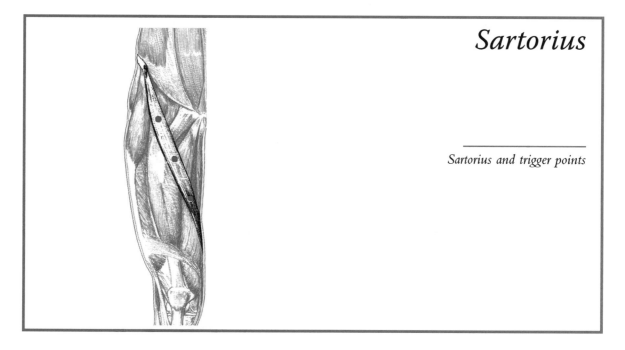

Sartorius

Sartorius and trigger points

SARTORIUS, the longest muscle in the body, is sometimes called the tailor sitting muscle. Sartorius attaches to the bony prominence on the front of the pelvis, your hip bone. It crosses the thigh to attach to the inside of the knee below the knee joint. When it contracts it works with other muscles to flex, abduct, and externally rotate the thigh and to flex the knee. Its combined actions allow us to sit cross-legged on the floor, tailor style.

Trigger points develop in sartorius when trigger points in other muscles produce a referred pain pattern over the area of the thigh where sartorius is located. When trigger points are present you will experience a burst of sharp or tingling pain on the surface of your thigh along the course of the muscle. Trigger points can develop anywhere throughout the length of this muscle, and as a result the pain can be felt anywhere throughout the muscle.

To locate sartorius, sit on a chair and place your hand on the bony hip bone on the front of your pelvis just above the crease between your thigh and your torso. Move your hand down slightly toward the groin and then rotate your knee to the outside. You'll feel the contraction of sartorius as you do this movement. Trace the course of the muscle from the hip over the inside of the thigh and to the bottom of the knee joint, feeling for areas of tenderness. It's easiest to release trigger points in sartorius by simple finger pressure. Hold each position for several seconds until you feel the softening of the point under your fingers.

Stretching sartorius is most effectively accomplished at the same time as treatment. The localized pressure will produce an effective local stretch to the muscle.

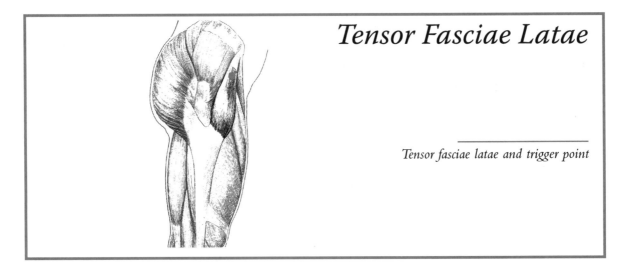

Tensor Fasciae Latae

Tensor fasciae latae and trigger point

TENSOR FASCIAE LATAE is a small, thick muscle that lies on the side of the pelvis. It attaches to the tibia, the larger of the two lower leg bones, through the long, thin, flat iliotibial band that runs along the outside of your thigh. It acts with other muscles to flex, abduct, and internally rotate the thigh. It helps to stabilize both the pelvis and the knee during walking and running.

Runners and walkers, particularly those who run on sloped or crowned roads, are at risk for developing trigger points in tensor fasciae latae. Jogging, running, or hiking up or down steep slopes may also create trigger points here, particularly if footgear does not provide adequate support. Lying in the fetal position or sitting for long periods of time with your knees higher than your hips can be a source of difficulty for this muscle as well. When trigger points are present in tensor fasciae latae, pain is felt deep in the hip at the area of the greater trochanter, the bony upper end of the long thigh bone. Pain may run down the outside of the thigh toward the knee. You may not be able to sit for long periods of time without pain and walking rapidly may be difficult. Because of tenderness at the greater trochanter, trigger points in this muscle can be easily mistaken for trochanteric bursitis.

To find tensor fasciae latae, lie on your back. Place your hand on the outside of your hip bone. When you press your knees together you should feel the contraction of tensor fasciae latae on the outside of your pelvis. Massage through its fibers to locate taut bands and tender spots. To release them, roll over onto your side and place a small, hard ball between the muscle and the floor. Let the weight of your body compress the trigger points against the ball.

Stretch tensor fasciae latae after you've worked on it. Stand or sit on the edge of a chair. Flex your leg and grasp the ankle with your hand. Rotate your knee outwardly just a bit as you extend your hip and bring your foot up toward your buttock. Hold the stretch for a good count of fifteen to twenty. Repeat this several times a day for a complete release.

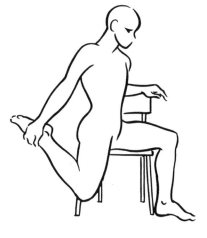

Stretch: Tensor fasciae latae

Thigh and Knee Pain

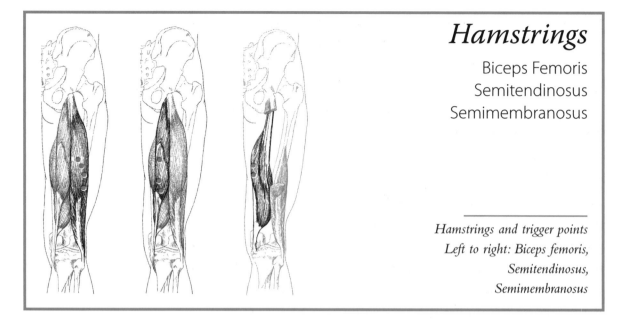

Hamstrings

Biceps Femoris
Semitendinosus
Semimembranosus

Hamstrings and trigger points
Left to right: Biceps femoris,
Semitendinosus,
Semimembranosus

TIGHTNESS OF THE HAMSTRINGS, the muscles that lie on the back of the thigh, is a common source of difficulty for athletes and non-athletes alike. It is the most frequent reason that people are unable to touch their toes in a forward-bending position. Hamstring tightness contributes to the flattening of the normal lumbar curve and to tightness in the muscles of the low back. Hamstring tightness is as common in children as it is in adults.

You can judge for yourself whether your hamstrings are tight. Lie on your back with your legs extended. Lift one leg as high off the floor as you can, keeping both knees straight and your low back on the floor; keep your neck and upper shoulders relaxed. You should be able to aim your toes just about straight up to the ceiling: 80 degrees is "normal."★ Anything less than that, or if you need to bend your knees or arch your back to bring your leg up, tells you that you've got tight hamstrings.

The hamstring muscles are "two-joint" muscles: they cross the hip *and* the knee and therefore act on both. There are three hamstring muscles: biceps femoris, semitendinosus, and semimembranosus. They all attach to the pelvis at the ischial tuberosities, the sitz bones. Biceps femoris attaches below the knee joint to the knobby head of the fibula, the smaller of the two lower leg bones. Semitendinosus and semimembranosus attach below the knee joint, one on top of the other, on the inside of the leg to the back of the tibia, the larger of the two lower leg bones.

Thigh and Knee Pain

■

★Kendall, McCreary, and Provance, 36.

The hamstring muscles flex the lower leg (bringing the heel toward the buttock) and extend the thigh, a movement that helps in stair climbing and is essential in keeping the trunk upright. The hamstrings help to prevent you from falling forward while walking.

Compression of the hamstrings often is the source of trigger points. Sitting on a chair or in a car where the seat presses into the back of the thighs is a recipe for hamstring trigger points. Overloading the muscle during sports activities that involve running will produce trigger points: football, basketball, and soccer are such sports. Keeping the hamstrings in the shortened position will produce trigger points—riding an ill-fitted bicycle, practicing poor technique while swimming, taking lengthy hikes or walks down steep hills, and a long period of bed rest all keep the hamstrings in a shortened position for an extended time.

When trigger points are present in biceps femoris, pain will be felt at the back of the outside of the knee; with trigger points in semitendinosus and semimembranosus, pain will be felt in the lower part of the buttock and the upper part of the thigh. Pain may extend down into the back of the thigh and the leg as far as the calf. You may have pain while walking, so much so that you might even be limping. Sitting is very uncomfortable; compression of the thighs against the chair seat exacerbates the pain. It's no wonder that hamstring trigger points are often mistaken for sciatica. Because the hamstrings work so closely with the quadriceps, trigger points in the hamstrings will also produce a considerable strain on the quads. This could lead to pain in the front of the thighs and knees. This pain won't be resolved until the tightness in both the hamstrings and the quads is resolved.

You can feel the attachments of the hamstrings while you're sitting down. Their upper attachment is on the ischial tuberosities, the sitz bones. If you place your hands, palms up, under your buttocks when you are sitting on a chair and then shift your hips back and forth a bit you will feel the sitz bones move. To feel the lower attachment of the hamstrings, hold on to your right knee with your right hand around the outside and your left hand around the inside. Place your fingertips into the hollow at the back of your knee. That's the popliteal space. With your hands in this position, your right hand can feel the tendon of biceps femoris and your left hand can feel the tendon of semitendinosus (the tendon of semismembranosus lies beneath semitendinosus, so you won't be able to feel it).

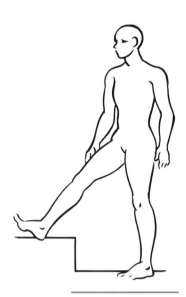

Stretch 1: Hamstrings

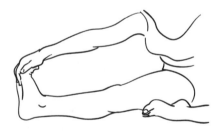

Stretch 2: Hamstrings

You can work on hamstring trigger points either seated in a chair or sitting on the floor with your leg extended in front of you. Place a small, hard ball such as a tennis ball underneath your thigh at the area of greatest tenderness, most likely in the midpoint of your thigh, either to the left or to the right of center, depending on which hamstring is most affected. Let the compression of the muscle work to elongate taut bands of muscle and release the trigger points. Keep at this. Treat all the trigger points in the hamstrings for a complete release.

Stretch the hamstrings following treatment. Place the heel of the leg to be stretched on a step, a ledge, or a chair seat. Make sure that your thigh is directly in front of your hips, not off to the side, and that your toes are pointing straight up. Maintain the angle between your hip and your thigh as you slowly bend forward from the hips. Your leg does not have to be high up to feel the stretch. If the position of your hip and thigh is correct you will feel a great stretch. Hold this for a good count of fifteen to twenty and repeat it regularly throughout the day.

You can also stretch the hamstrings by sitting on the floor with your leg extended in front of you. You can do this one leg at a time or both legs at the same time. Keeping your knee straight, place the palm of your hand on the bottom of your foot. Pull your toes and your ankle toward you. Hold this position for a good count of fifteen to twenty.

Once you've eliminated your pain through self-treatment and stretching, it's important to work on lengthening the hamstrings to avoid all the pitfalls that shortened hamstrings can bring. You will have to be patient and consistent with the stretching—it may take weeks or months for true lengthening but it is so important that it's worth the time and the effort. Because of the close working relationship between the adductors (page 130) and the hamstrings, it is extremely important to stretch your adductors in addition to your hamstrings to get a complete release. See the adductor stretch on page 131 for instructions.

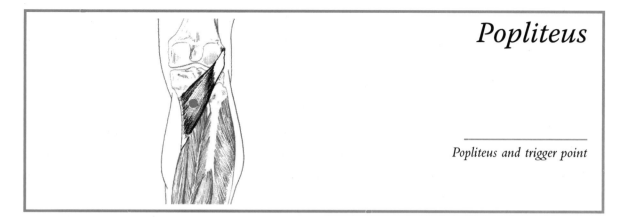

Popliteus

Popliteus and trigger point

POPLITEUS is a small muscle that lies in the back of the knee. It attaches to the outside of the thigh bone and to the tibia, the longer of the two lower leg bones. It aids in bending the knees by helping to unlock the knee joint. It also helps to prevent the forward movement of the thigh on the lower leg when you crouch or place your weight on a bent knee.

Trigger points can develop in popliteus during sports that require quick starts, stops, and twists with the knees bent—downhill skiers, hikers, tennis players, soccer players, football players, ice skaters, and dancers can all be at risk. So can women who wear high heels. Trigger points develop in popliteus in combination with trigger points in the hamstrings and gastrocnemius. Once those trigger points are released the popliteus trigger points become apparent.

Popliteal trigger points cause pain in the back of the knee, particularly when crouching, running or walking downhill, or going down stairs. You may not be able to straighten your knee without pain.

Popliteus is difficult to work on because it lies in the back of the knee underneath the top end of the two large calf muscles—gastrocnemius and soleus. Sit on a chair and place your bent leg on a footstool. Place your fingers in the back of your knee. You'll feel sharp tendons on the back of the inside of the knee. Massage deeply just beside those tendons through the thick muscle that lies next to them. Work with your fingers, even though they may get tired. There are too many delicate structures in the back of your knee that can be harmed by using a harder object there.

Stretching popliteus is done sitting in a low chair with your foot on the ground, or at a common height with your leg on a footstool. Flex your lower leg 15 to 20 degrees. Hold on to the lower end of your thigh to prevent your thigh from moving as you rotate your lower leg to the outside. You will feel as though you're hardly moving, but rest assured that the muscle is being stretched. Hold this for a count of fifteen to twenty and repeat the stretch two or three times each session.

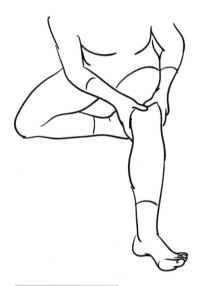

Stretch: Popliteus

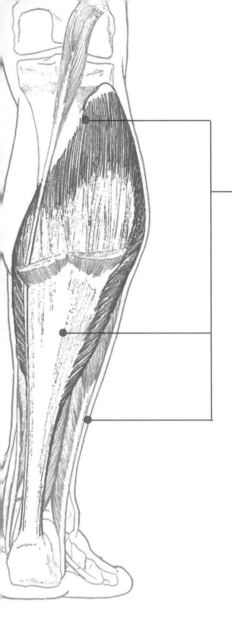

Lower Leg, Ankle, and Foot Pain

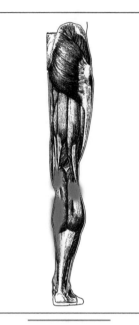

Pain pattern: Gastrocnemius

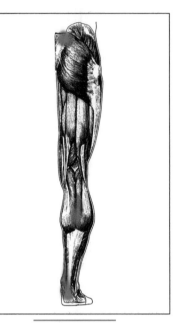

Pain pattern: Soleus

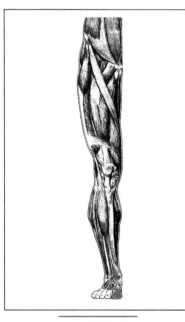

Pain pattern: Tibialis anterior

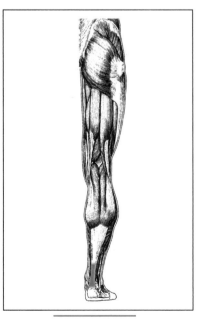

Pain pattern: Tibialis posterior

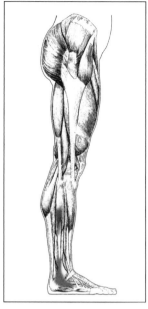

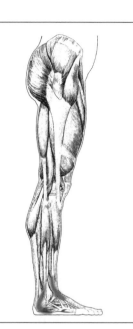

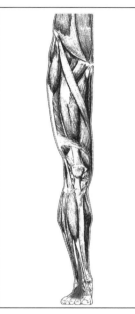

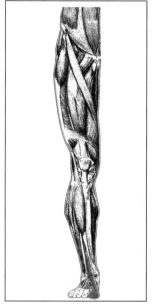

Peroneus longus and
Peroneus brevis

Peroneus tertius

Extensor digitorum
longus

Extensor hallucis
longus

Pain pattern: Peroneals

Pain pattern: Long extensors of the toes

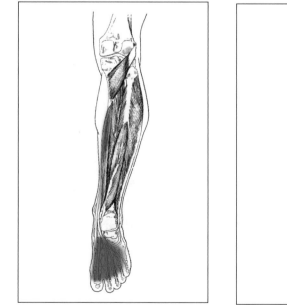

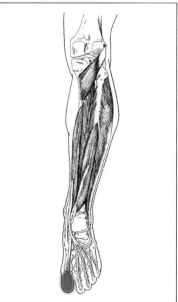

Flexor digitorum longus

Flexor hallucis longus

Pain pattern: Long flexors of the toes

Running, jogging, jumping, sprinting, walking, hiking, kicking, leaping, dancing: what do all of these activities have in common?

Each in its own way may be a source of injury to the muscles and joints of the foot and leg.

Twenty-eight bones form the leg, ankle, and foot. The ankle and foot consist of seven tarsal bones, five metatarsal bones, and the fourteen phalanges that comprise the bony structure of the five toes. Our ability to stand, balance, walk, and take part in the activities that we love hinges on the proper function of this part of the body. The lower leg, ankle, and foot provide the base of support necessary for our upright posture. This part of our bodies bears our weight and suffers our bad landings and shoe choices.

Ankle sprains are among the most common injuries in sports. Landing from a jump or leap on the side of the foot, stepping on a loose rock, stepping off a curb on a misplaced foot—all of these activities and more can lead to an ankle sprain and injury to those muscles that act on the ankle and foot. The peroneal muscles are particularly impacted by a twist of the ankle. It is unfortunately the case that they are often overlooked in the treatment of a sprained ankle.

The dancer, the gymnast, and the martial artist use the feet to perform complicated combinations of movements in which balance is critical, balance that must emanate from the feet. Their actions depend on the strength and integrated action of the muscles of their lower legs and feet. And yet it is just these actions that may be the source of overuse injuries to those very critical muscles. The legs and feet are the foundation of activity for runners, joggers, walkers, and hikers; the legs and feet receive the brunt of uneven or hard surfaces, soft sandy beaches, and ungroomed trails and hills. Basketball players, tennis players, and hurdlers jump—and land—over and over again. Soccer players, football players, and baseball players run and kick, start, stop, and turn "on a dime."

In some sports the use of the feet and lower legs is obvious; in others it is less so. Alpine skiers strap their feet and ankles in boots

> **Cautionary Statement**
>
> A severe injury needs immediate medical attention. Please consult with your physician in the event of the following:
>
> - an acute injury with severe pain
> - bleeding, bruising, or joint deformity
> - sudden painful swelling and the inability to bend the ankle, foot, or toes
> - inability to support the body's weight on the injured leg
> - pain, tenderness, redness, swelling, and/or fever

that prevent their freedom of movement and may stay in those boots for hours on end. This is essential in downhill skiing. Yet this very immobility may be the source of the development of trigger points in some of the muscles of the lower leg.

Athletics and dance is not the only source of injury to the muscles of the legs and feet. Ill-fitting footwear or footwear that is worn and fails to provide adequate support and stability is a common source of injuries to the muscles of the legs and feet. The internal support structure of sports shoes frequently wears out before the shoe appears to be old and worn on the outside. Women often select shoes following the fashion of the day, some of which may not provide sufficient stability for the foot. Whether it is a heel that is too high, a toe that is too pointed, or a shoe that easily slides off the foot, walking in such shoes, even for a short distance, can lead to strains in the muscles of the legs and feet.

Improper, ill-fitting, or inadequate footwear may adversely effect more than just the muscles of the feet, ankles and legs. Proper support of the lower limb is essential for proper alignment of the knees, hips, and back. Lack of support may lead to pain and dysfunction in these areas and may act to delay or inhibit complete healing of the muscles in these areas, should problems arise there.

The feet are the foundation for our upright posture. Regardless of your profession, your passions, or your avocation, becoming aware of the importance of maintaining a stable foundation is an important part of reducing muscle restrictions and injuries to the feet and legs, as well as the knees, hips, and back.

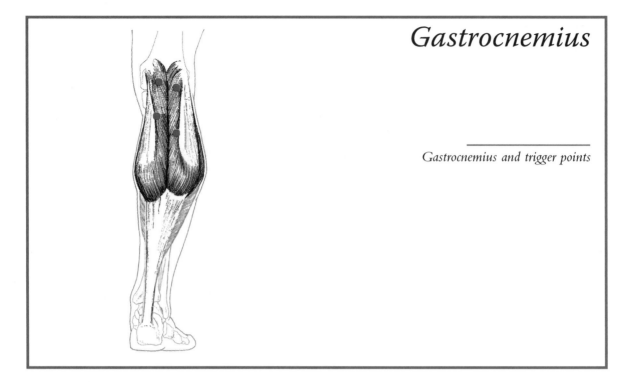

Gastrocnemius

Gastrocnemius and trigger points

THE GASTROCNEMIUS is the muscle that gives the calf its characteristic shape. It has two muscular heads, or bellies, that lie on the upper two-thirds of the lower leg. The upper fibers of gastrocnemius attach to the femur (the long thigh bone), cross the knee joint, and then join with the soleus muscle to attach to the back of the heel through the Achilles tendon. The primary action of the gastrocnemius is to plantarflex the foot, the action that you do when you point your foot or stand on the ball of your foot. Because its upper fibers cross the knee joint, it also helps to flex the knee when the leg is not supporting the body's weight.

Trigger points develop in gastrocnemius due to overloading the muscle: pointing the foot too much and too hard (excessive plantarflexion). Dancers, and particularly ballet dancers—who continuously work to develop a strongly pointed foot with a beautiful arch so that they can dance on a high demi-pointe—are at continual risk for trigger points here. Women who wear high-heeled shoes are at risk. Swimmers and divers may also develop trigger points in the gastrocnemius because of the plantarflexed position of their feet when they swim or dive. Activities that involve working the muscle while it is in a stretched position can be equally problematic: jogging uphill, climbing steep slopes, or walking up slanted surfaces. Those cyclists who ride on ill-fitted bicycles are also at risk for developing trigger points here. If the seat is too low the gastrocnemius is overworked

Lower Leg, Ankle, and
Foot Pain

while pedaling. Immobility of the leg and reduced leg circulation also contribute to trigger point development in the muscle.

When there are trigger points in gastrocnemius, pain is most often experienced locally in the calf. In some cases pain may radiate to the back of the knee and possibly to the instep as well. Trigger points will not produce noticeably restricted motion or weakness in the muscle. However, you may not be able to fully straighten your knee when your foot is flexed with your toes pulled back (a position called dorsiflexion). Trigger points may also produce calf cramps at night during hours of sleep.

Because there are two bellies of gastrocnemius, you will need to palpate both to identify taut bands and trigger points. Sit on the floor with your leg extended in front of you, your knee bent, and your foot relaxed on the floor. You can also sit on a couch or chair and place your foot on a footstool or coffee table in front of you. If you are working on your right leg, your right hand will work on the belly on the outer side of the leg and your left hand will work on the belly on the inner side. If it's easier you can work on one muscle belly at a time.

Feel the back of your heel. Attaching to it is the thickest and strongest tendon in the body, the Achilles tendon. Palpate the tendon up toward the middle of your calf. You'll be able to feel the difference in texture where the thick tendon merges with the softer, more supple muscle. Continue working up the muscle toward the back of the knee, feeling for taut bands and tender spots within those bands. Once you've found the bands, use your fingers, a pencil eraser, or any of the treatment devices available on the market to compress the trigger point. Trigger points in gastrocnemius take a lot of work—several sessions a day for several days in a row—in order to release completely. And stretching the muscle is essential after working on it.

To stretch gastrocnemius, place the ball of your foot on a step or curb and allow the heel of the foot to drop below the level of the step. Keep the knee straight as you stretch the calf. Hold this position for a count of twenty-five to thirty.

You can also stand approximately 12 inches from a wall, placing your hands on the wall at chest level. Place the leg to be stretched approximately 18 inches behind the other leg, making sure to keep the toes of both feet facing the wall and the feet hip-width apart. Bend the front knee, keeping the rear leg straight. Your weight should remain on the front leg. Hold this position for a count of twenty-five to thirty.

Stretch gastrocnemius many times a day for a complete release.

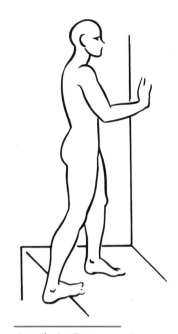

Stretch 1: Gastrocnemius

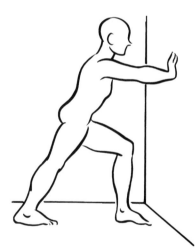

Stretch 2: Gastrocnemius

Lower Leg, Ankle, and
Foot Pain
■

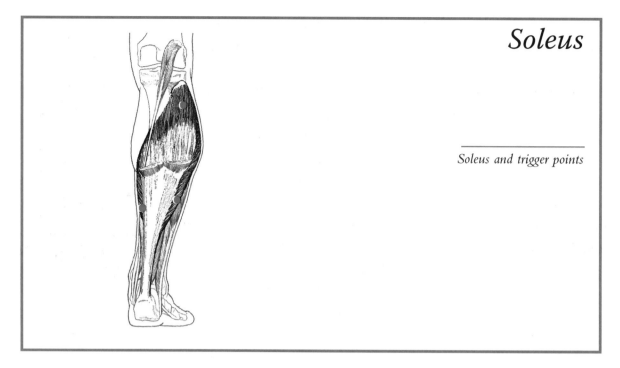

Soleus

Soleus and trigger points

THE SOLEUS MUSCLE lies just underneath the gastrocnemius. Its upper fibers connect to both bones of the lower leg: the tibia (the larger of the two bones) and the fibula (the smaller outside bone). Soleus joins with gastrocnemius to attach to the heel through the Achilles tendon. Soleus works to plantarflex the foot, the action that you do when you point your foot or stand on the ball of your foot. It also works to provide stability to the ankle joint.

Trigger points develop in soleus primarily through muscle overload. Dancers moving on a floor that is too slippery are at risk for soleus trigger points, as is any one of us when walking on icy sidewalks or wet floors. Walking or jogging on a slanted surface or a crowned road will also overload soleus and lead to trigger points. Landing on the ball of your foot while dancing, jumping, leaping, or jogging can lead to trigger points. So can hiking up steep hills. Skating or skiing without sufficient ankle support may also lead to trigger points in soleus.

When trigger points are present in the lower part of the muscle on the inside of the leg, the most common complaint is heel pain and tenderness. Not only will you experience pain throughout the course of the Achilles tendon, but the heel itself may be quite tender to the touch. You may not be able to dorsiflex (flex) your foot fully without pain due to the restriction caused by the trigger points. This can lead to difficulty walking, especially up hills or up and down stairs. These symptoms might lead to a diagnosis of Achilles tendinitis; however, releasing the trigger points will eliminate the pain and symptoms. Less commonly, trigger points can develop on the outer side of the leg in the middle of the muscle, causing pain in the center of the calf. Most atypical is the trigger point in the upper part of the muscle, which causes pain in the center of the low back at the juncture of the sacrum and the pelvis (the sacroiliac joint).

To locate the most common soleus trigger points, sit in a chair and place the ankle of the leg to be worked over your other knee. First identify the thick Achilles tendon attaching at the heel. Palpate the tendon up toward the middle of the calf and identify where it attaches to the more supple musculature of the gastrocnemius (page 156). Place your thumb at the juncture of the Achilles tendon and the gastrocnemius. Move your thumb around toward the front of your leg and you will feel the back of the long leg bone, the tibia. The muscle that you feel between the Achilles tendon and the bone is the soleus.

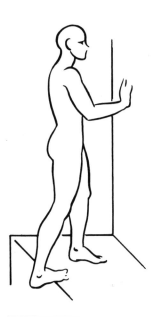

Stretch 1: Soleus

Trigger points will be located in taut bands lying between the tendon and the bone. This is the trigger point that causes heel pain. Using your thumb, palpate soleus to identify tender spots. Compress tender spots with your thumb until you feel a softening and a release under your finger. Repeat this several times through the day to completely release the muscle.

To find trigger points in the upper part of the muscle, place your foot on a footstool or coffee table. Feel the upper part of the outside of your lower leg, just underneath your knee joint. Here you will feel the round bony head of the fibula, the smaller of the two lower leg bones. Palpate deeply for taut bands and trigger points lying underneath the head of the fibula. This trigger point causes mid-calf pain. Follow those bands about halfway down the leg to find trigger points on the outer side of soleus. These trigger points cause the unusual symptom of pain in the low back at the juncture of the sacrum and the pelvis. To completely release the muscle you'll have to work on these trigger points several times throughout the day.

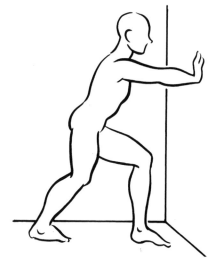

Stretch 2: Soleus

Follow up treatment with stretching. Stretch soleus by placing the ball of the foot on a step or curb. Allow the heel of the foot to drop below the level of the step. Keep your knee bent as you stretch the calf. Hold the position for a count of twenty-five to thirty.

You can also stand approximately 12 inches from a wall, placing your hands on the wall at chest level. Place the leg to be stretched approximately 18 inches behind the other, making sure to keep the toes of both feet facing the wall and the feet hip-width apart. Bend both knees to stretch soleus. Hold this position for a count of twenty-five to thirty.

Lower Leg, Ankle, and
Foot Pain

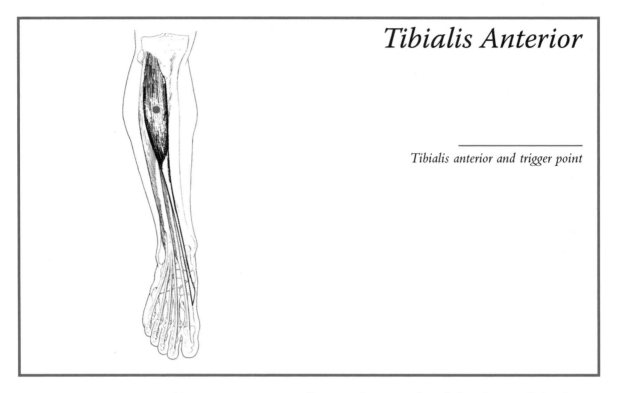

Tibialis Anterior

Tibialis anterior and trigger point

TIBIALIS ANTERIOR lies on the outside of the front of the lower leg, right next to your shin. It attaches to the upper part of the large lower leg bone, the tibia. Its fibers lie in the upper two-thirds of the space between the tibia and the fibula (the smaller of the lower leg bones). Its tendon crosses to the inside of your ankle and attaches to the bottom of your foot just about at the center of your arch.

Tibialis anterior dorsiflexes the foot (bringing the top of your foot toward your shin) and inverts the foot. To invert your foot, place it flat on the floor. Lift the arch and big toe off the floor, keeping the blade of your foot, the pinky side, on the floor. (Eversion is the opposite action. To evert your foot, place it on the floor and lift the blade of your foot, keeping your big toe and your arch down.)

Tibialis anterior helps to maintain balance while you are standing. It is highly active during most sports and dance endeavors, especially fast walking, running, jogging, sprinting, and jumping upward from two feet. Basketball players and dancers would seem to be at great risk for trigger points in tibialis anterior.

Trigger points most commonly develop in tibialis anterior as a result of trauma to the ankle joint, such as an ankle sprain or fracture. However, walking on a rough surface or on a crowned road can affect the muscle as well. Tightness in the two large calf muscles, the gastrocnemius and soleus, can also lead to restriction of tibialis anterior. Think about how this might impact dancers. Ballet dancers are always trying to master a high demi-pointe and strong arch, actions that consistently tighten the gastrocnemius and soleus, and they are regularly doing upward jumps from two feet. Both are primary sources of trigger points in tibialis anterior.

When there are trigger points in tibialis anterior, pain will be felt mostly at the inside of the front of your ankle and your big toe. There may be some pain on the outside of the leg where the muscle lies. You might feel that your ankle is weak and you might trip or fall because your toes aren't clearing the floor when you walk.

To locate tibialis anterior you'll have to find your shin, which is actually part of your tibia. The upper part of your shin can be felt just underneath your knee. Its sharp edge can be felt throughout the length of your lower leg. Tibialis anterior lies just on the outer side of the shin. Begin palpating it just underneath your knee. Massage down the outside of your lower leg just beside your shin, remembering that tibialis anterior only lies on the upper two-thirds of your lower leg. Massage deeply to locate taut bands. Trigger points are frequently found about one-third of the way down the muscle, but they can develop anywhere along its length, so palpate the muscle thoroughly. You can see where the tendon crosses your ankle joint if you dorsiflex (flex) and invert your foot. The tendon pops right out on the top of the inside of your ankle.

To stretch tibialis anterior, point your foot as strongly as you can and cross it over the ankle of your standing leg so that your toes are pointing away from your body and your heel is pointing up toward the ceiling. Bend the knee of your standing leg into the back of the knee of the leg you are stretching. Hold this position for a count of twenty-five to thirty. As with other muscles of the lower leg, you'll have to repeatedly stretch tibialis anterior throughout the day in order to obtain complete release. You'll also have to stretch the gastrocnemius (page 157) and soleus (page 159) muscles to release your lower leg completely.

Stretch: Tibialis anterior

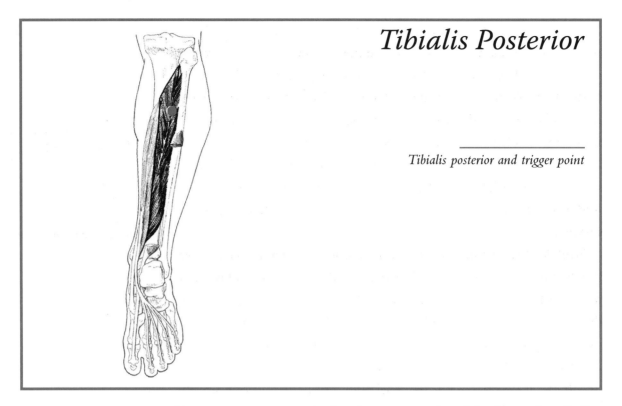

Tibialis Posterior

Tibialis posterior and trigger point

TIBIALIS POSTERIOR is the deepest muscle of the lower leg. It lies deep underneath soleus, attaching to the rear surfaces of the two lower leg bones, the tibia and the fibula. Its tendon passes behind the inner ankle bone to attach on the bottom of the foot to most of the bones that form the arch of the foot. Tibialis posterior keeps the weight balanced evenly on the foot, preventing too much weight from dropping into the arch while you're walking. It distributes the weight of the body evenly among the bones of the foot.

Trigger points in tibialis posterior most frequently develop when other muscles of the lower leg are involved; it is rarely involved in isolation. However, jogging on uneven surfaces or crowned roads, foot weakness, and wearing badly worn shoes that don't provide support against rocking of the foot can contribute to trigger point development.

Trigger points here will produce severe pain over the Achilles tendon above the heel as well as in the sole of the foot, particularly the arch. There may be some pain over the middle of the calf, at the heel, and in the bottom of the foot and the toes. Walking or running, particularly on uneven surfaces, may be very painful. If tibialis posterior has had trigger points for a long time, when you walk it might appear that your arch has dropped and you have become flat-footed.

Because of its deep location in the calf, tibialis posterior can't be

Lower Leg, Ankle, and
Foot Pain

directly palpated, but you can get a sense of its soreness through the overlying musculature. Sit with the ankle of your painful leg crossed over your other knee. Find your shin with your fingertips. Work your fingers over the hard tibia toward the back of your leg, feeling for the place where the bone stops and soft muscle begins. That's the back of the tibia. Use your thumbs to press into the back of the tibia in the upper one-half of your leg. If there are trigger points present, soreness will be felt about halfway between your knee fold and the midpoint of your lower leg. Use your thumbs to massage into that soreness.

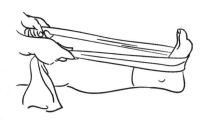

Stretch: Tibialis posterior

Stretch tibialis posterior sitting on the floor with your leg extended in front of you. Place a towel or dynaband around the ball of your foot and pull your foot toward you. Pull with a bit more force on the blade of your foot (the little toe side). This will lift the blade of the foot a bit, everting it. Hold the stretch for a count of fifteen to twenty. Repeat several times throughout the day.

If there are trigger points in tibialis posterior there will be trigger points in the other lower leg muscles as well. Make sure you stretch them all for complete release.

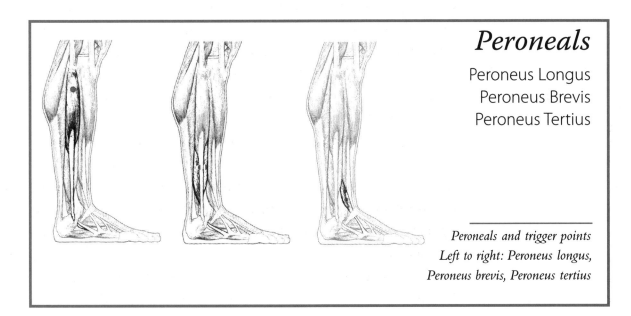

Peroneals
Peroneus Longus
Peroneus Brevis
Peroneus Tertius

Peroneals and trigger points
Left to right: Peroneus longus,
Peroneus brevis, Peroneus tertius

THE LONG, THIN PERONEAL MUSCLES lie on the outside of your lower leg. Peroneus longus attaches to the top of the fibula on the side of your knee. Peroneus brevis attaches to the lower two-thirds of the fibula and lies underneath longus. Together their long tendons pass behind the outer ankle bone and attach to the middle of the

Lower Leg, Ankle, and
Foot Pain

blade of your foot. Peroneus tertius attaches to the lower one-half of the front of the fibula. Its tendon passes in front of the outer anklebone and attaches with the other two peroneal muscles to the middle of the blade of the foot.

The peroneals are the primary evertors of the foot. They bring the blade of the foot off the floor.

Trigger points develop in the peroneal muscles by twisting or spraining your ankle, particularly when you fall off your foot in such a way as to land on the blade of your foot. Ankle sprains are among the most common injuries in sports. Runners, joggers, dancers, basketball players, gymnasts, tennis players: every athlete is at risk. Immobility of the ankle and foot is another means by which trigger points develop. If an injury requires that you need to use a cast, peroneal trigger points may develop. Trigger points may also develop when tibialis anterior or tibialis posterior are chronically tight. Wearing high heels, crossing the legs at the knees, and having flat feet all may lead to trigger points here.

Ankle pain and tenderness with ankle weakness or instability are primary symptoms of peroneal trigger points. Ankle pain is usually right around the outer anklebone with some pain spreading through to the blade of the foot. When the pain is around the outside of the anklebone peroneus longus and brevis are usually the source; when the pain is in front of the anklebone peroneus tertius is usually the source. Tenderness due to trigger points can be differentiated from an ankle sprain, the injury to a ligament so common in sports. An ankle sprain usually is accompanied by swelling of the ankle and pain that is focused right at the outer side of the ankle joint. When trigger points are the source of the pain there won't be any ankle swelling and the pain will be more generalized throughout the ankle.

To locate the peroneals you'll first have to identify the upper part of the fibula, the smaller of the two long bones in the lower leg. Place your hand on the outer side of your knee joint. Feel for a small bony knob just underneath the joint. That's the upper part of the fibula. Use your fingertips to trace the sharp edge of the fibula all the way down the side of your lower leg to the bone on the outside of your ankle. The knob on the top of your leg is the top of the fibula; the bone on the outside of the ankle is its lower part. The peroneals lie along the front margin of that bone.

Palpate the peroneals just in front of the fibula. If you evert your foot at the same time—lift the blade of your foot off the floor—you'll feel the contraction of the muscles under your fingers. When trigger points are present you'll feel the muscles as taut bands. The peroneus longus trigger point can be felt about 1 inch below the knob at the top of the fibula; the peroneus brevis trigger points can be felt approximately two-thirds of the way down the leg. Palpate in front of the lower ankle bone in order to feel peroneus tertius and its trigger point. Keep everting your foot to make sure that you are following the bands of the peroneals.

To stretch the peroneals, sit with your leg extended in front of you. Place a strap or towel around your foot. Use the opposite arm to pull the foot gently, allowing it to dorsiflex (flex) and rotate inwardly. You will feel the stretch on the outside of your leg. Hold the position for a count of fifteen to twenty. Repeat this several times throughout the day for a complete release.

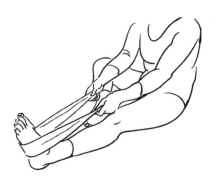

Stretch: Peroneals

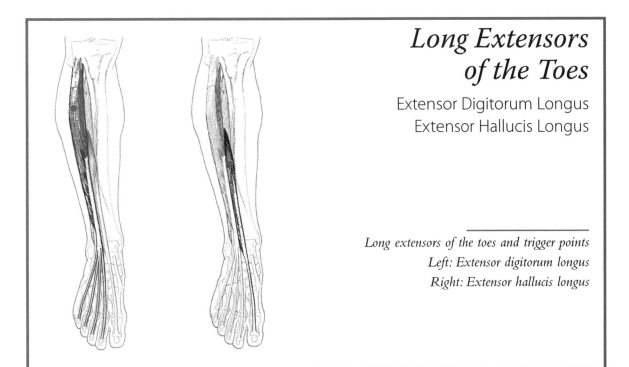

Long Extensors of the Toes
Extensor Digitorum Longus
Extensor Hallucis Longus

Long extensors of the toes and trigger points
Left: Extensor digitorum longus
Right: Extensor hallucis longus

THE LONG EXTENSORS, extensor digitorum longus and extensor hallucis longus, work together to extend all the toes. Both of them assist other muscles to dorsiflex the foot, pulling the top of the foot toward the leg. The long extensors lie in the space between the tibia and the fibula. After crossing the ankle, extensor digitorum longus attaches to the four small toes. Extensor hallucis longus attaches to

Lower Leg, Ankle, and
Foot Pain

■

the end of the big toe. Efficient functioning of these muscles is essential for the proper working of the foot during standing and walking. Both muscles work strongly in a standing jump.

Trigger points develop in the long extensors through muscular overload. Walking in soft sand or walking or jogging on uneven or crowned roads can be a source, as can tripping or falling. Wearing high-heeled shoes can contribute to their injury, as can practicing dance on a strong demi-pointe. Immobilization of the leg and foot, as happens in wearing a cast, can be another source of difficulty for the long extensors.

When trigger points are present in extensor digitorum longus, pain is experienced at the top of the foot and the three middle toes. Sometimes the pain may be felt up into the ankle and possibly up into the lower one-half of the lower leg. Trigger points in extensor hallucis longus will produce pain in the big toe and possibly into the ankle. You might experience night cramps along the course of these muscles if trigger points are present; the existence of taut bands and trigger points over a long time may cause hammertoes to develop.

To locate extensor digitorum longus you'll first have to find tibialis anterior, just beside the shin (page 160), and peroneus longus, just in front of the fibula (page 163). Once you've found these muscles you can palpate extensor digitorum longus between them. Taut bands can be felt about 3 inches down from the knobby upper end of the fibula. Extensor hallucis longus lies between tibialis anterior and extensor digitorum longus throughout the upper two-thirds of the lower leg. You can locate it just below the level of the lower one-third of the lower leg in front of the fibula. Once you've located the taut bands you can press directly into the muscle with your fingers or treatment device.

Stretching of the long extensors is essential. In the standing position, place a strongly pointed foot across the ankle of your standing leg. Place the toes of the leg to be stretched beside the heel of the standing leg. Bend the knee of the standing leg into the back of the knee of the bent leg to stretch the top of your foot. Hold this position for a good count of fifteen to twenty. Repeat this many times through the day for a complete release.

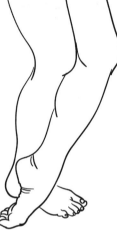

Stretch: Long extensors of the toes

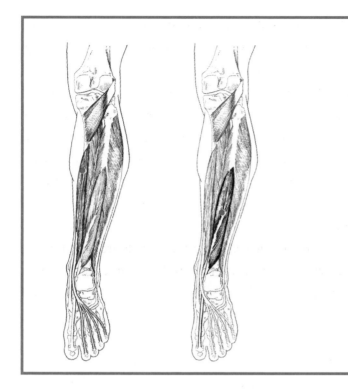

Long Flexors of the Toes

Flexor Digitorum Longus
Flexor Hallucis Longus

Long flexors of the toes and trigger points
Left: Flexor digitorum longus
Right: Flexor hallucis longus

THE LONG FLEXORS, flexor digitorum longus and flexor hallucis longus, together act to plantarflex (point) all the toes.

Flexor digitorum longus is a very deep muscle lying underneath the gastrocnemius and the soleus on the back of the calf. It attaches to the back of the tibia, runs the length of the lower leg, crosses behind the inner ankle bone, and attaches to each of the four small toes on the bottom of the foot. Flexor hallucis longus lies on the back of the fibula. It runs down the back of the lower leg, crosses behind the inner ankle bone, and attaches to the bottom of the big toe. Together these two muscles help to maintain balance when the weight of the body is on the front of the foot. They help to stabilize the ankle while walking. Both of these muscles are extremely active during take off and landing in a vertical two-legged jump.

Trigger points can develop in these long flexors by running on uneven ground, soft sand, or crowned surfaces, or as a function of wearing shoes that do not provide adequate support in the sole of the foot or the heel. Wearing shoes that are not sufficiently flexible may also produce trigger points. When trigger points develop in flexor digitorum longus, pain will be experienced in the middle of the sole of the foot and possibly over the bottom surface of the four small toes. With trigger points in flexor hallucis longus, pain will be experienced in the bottom of the big toe and the ball of the foot

Lower Leg, Ankle, and
Foot Pain

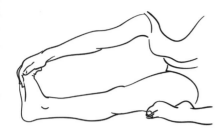

Stretch: Long flexors of the toes

adjacent to it. Pain will be worse while standing. Hammertoes may develop as a result of taut bands in these muscles.

Because of the placement of these muscles underneath the gastrocnemius and the soleus, it is difficult to feel the long flexors. To locate trigger points in flexor digitorum longus, sit on a chair and cross the ankle of your painful foot over the knee of the other leg. Find the sharp edge of the tibia, the shin. Move your hand across its hard surface toward the back of your leg. Here you'll be able to feel the back surface of the tibia. Locate flexor digitorum longus about 3 inches below the knee joint, between the tibia and the bulky gastrocnemius. Press against the back of the tibia and then toward the outer side of the leg to feel tenderness in flexor digitorum longus. Flexor hallucis longus can't be directly palpated at all. You'll have to press through the thick soleus to get to it. Press deeply, using your thumb or treatment device, about two-thirds of the way down the leg from the knee joint. It will be just about where the Achilles tendon starts. Press in and toward the outside of the leg, toward the fibula, to feel tenderness from a restricted flexor hallucis longus.

Stretching is essential to really release the long flexors. Sit on the floor with your leg extended in front of you. Place the palm of your hand on the bottom of your foot, pulling your toes toward you. Let your ankle relax and it, too, will flex with the stretch. Hold this position for a good count of fifteen to twenty. Repeat this many times through the day for a complete release.

Guidelines for Injury Prevention

The most important action you can take to prevent injuries from occurring is to maintain your general health. Regardless of your age, your sport, your capabilities, or your "day job," making a habit of taking care of yourself is the easiest way to ensure a long, joyful participation in your physical endeavors of choice. What follows are a few simple guidelines that you can use to keep fit, reduce stress, and avoid injury. Think about them, consider them, modify them to fit your life, practice them as best you can. Live healthy and play hard!

Listen to your body.

The human body is a miraculous, intelligent machine. It is capable of healing itself. It has the capacity to alert us to its needs. Sometimes the way it alerts us is through pain, fatigue, cold, fever, headache, malaise, and dysfunction. The purpose of this feedback, of course, is to show us that there is a problem and that we need to behave in ways that will prevent the problem from getting worse. The usefulness of these signals, however, is limited by our willingness to pay attention to them and to heed the warning signs.

Athletes, and particularly adult athletes, are often passionate about their sport. We see it in the adult dancer, who will do just about anything to avoid missing a class, or golfers who are out on the golf course each time they can get out there regardless of weather or how they feel. We see this dedication in all sports and in many athletes. How many of us have chosen to work out even when we hurt a little or had a headache or had some kind of an injury that we were sure would go away? We see kids push through pain all the time. This was something that we, too, could easily get away with in our twenties and thirties. But once the forties and fifties come our resilience changes. We are more easily injured and it takes longer to heal. In our mature years it is especially important to listen to the body.

Be smart with yourself: Heed your body's warning signs. If you are particularly fatigued, skip your workout. If you are getting a cold or have the beginning signs of an upper respiratory ailment, don't push your way through a tough class. Doing so may well have the effect of bringing on the illness rather than burning it out. If your lower body muscles are particularly sore from yesterday's tough workout, stretch lightly and let them rest, even if you've planned to do a harder workout today. If you feel a bit of ankle soreness, don't run the long run today; instead, wait a couple of days to make sure your ankle is in the best shape it can be. Work with your body, *don't* fight with it.

Allow your body to rest when it needs rest. This is so very important. Practicing this one simple principle will go a long way in helping you avoid injury. Live in ways that let you continue to enjoy your body and your activities for a long time to come.

Warm up before you exercise.
Engaging in any sport or activity requires that our muscles be supple and elastic in order to move through the actions comfortably. Anyone who has engaged in any sport or physical activity knows how easily the muscles and joints can be injured when you aren't sufficiently warmed up. Every dancer knows that there is no way you can do jumps before preparing the legs, feet, hips, and back with a complete warm-up. As we age our muscles grow less supple and resilient. They tend toward shortening and tightening, which places greater stress on the joints. Engaging in physical activity without sufficient preparation of the muscle leaves both muscle and joint prone to injury. It is particularly important to prepare our muscles prior to engaging in activity, regardless of the activity that we are about to do.

It is generally a good idea to take a brief walk to warm the muscles. In addition, gentle, generalized stretching prior to muscular activity is a wonderful means of preparing the body for the work it is about to do. I cannot overstress the importance of the word *gentle* here. The aim of pre-exercise stretching is not to elongate the muscles but to bring blood and fluids into the muscle.

With this in mind, then, move about, put your joints through mild range-of-motion activities, walk. As you ready yourself for your sport, prepare your body for the work you're about to do, even if you don't consider it work!

Practice proper technique for your sport.
Proper technique is *so* important!

The easiest way to injure yourself while engaged in any sport is to use poor technique. Conversely, the best way to prevent injuries during the practice of any sport is to practice correct technique. Whatever your sport, study proper technique from the professionals. Take a class, or take a lesson; read books; practice properly. When our muscles were young and soft and supple we could get away with "fudging," but not any more. Now we really need to use our muscles properly. The rewards will be great—not only will your body work better, but your skill level in your sport will advance more rapidly than you can imagine.

Train throughout your day, not just during a workout.
A common piece of advice from fitness experts is that, in order to maintain optimal health, adults should engage in some form of physical exercise every day for at least thirty minutes. Between devoting hours to work and work-related activities; shopping, food preparation, cleaning, and errands to keep the home going; and hours devoted to the care of our children and / or our parents, there simply doesn't seem to be enough hours in the day to do everything we need to do, let alone all of the things we *want to do.*

That being said, it is still very important to do some form of exercise each day. So how do we accomplish that?

Getting exercise every day is really much simpler than it might appear to be. If you consider the forms that physical exercise takes, we can have several mini workouts throughout the day. To excel in any sport or activity the athlete needs to cross-train; every athlete needs to stretch and to develop strength, aerobic capacity, and balance. Rather than thinking about a daily workout as a time requirement, think about training your awareness. You need to *remember* throughout the day that what you want to do is physical training, even if you are not able to engage in your chosen sport.

For training when your time is tight, try implementing a few of the following suggestions:

1. Park your car a distance away from your destination and walk to get yourself there.

2. When you have the choice between the stairs or the elevator, walk the stairs. (Or walk just a few flights if the floor you need to get to is quite high up in the building.)

3. Take a break from your computer work and bend forward to stretch your back and legs. You can do this either seated or standing.

4. Stretch your neck when sitting on the train, in a car, in your living room.

5. When standing in the shower, stretch your back, legs, chest, and neck.

6. Stretch your sides and your back as you reach up to a high shelf.

7. When standing in line at the grocery store or at the bus stop, or when standing at the stove preparing food, place all your weight on one foot and balance.

8. Balance on one leg while you are putting on your pants, sock, or shoe.

9. To strengthen your arms and back, carry your groceries and other packages in your arms rather than in a bag over your shoulder.

10. Practice good posture throughout the day. This will help to develop strength in your back and torso. Elongate your head and neck as if the top of your head were suspended from the ceiling. Let the weight of your arms hanging at your sides stretch your shoulders down. Allow your shoulder blades to glide down toward your waist. Draw your lower ribs and your navel toward your spine without sucking in your lower belly. You can do this either seated or standing, at any and all times of the day, whenever you think of it.

11. Practice proper lifting techniques, regardless of the weight of the object to be lifted. Even if you are picking up something as light as a key, use your legs in the lift. Squat to bring your arms in reach of the object on the floor and use the force of your leg muscles to stand. Doing squats each time you pick something up from the floor will strengthen your legs and your back.

12. Relax your body. Systematically feel each part of your body, one part at a time. Get a sense of the tensions that are held in the muscles and intentionally relax them. Start with your face, jaw, head, and neck. Work your way into your shoulders, your arms and hands, your chest, upper back, and belly, and finally into your thighs, legs, and feet. You will be amazed at how much tension is locked in those muscles. Relaxing them will be a surprising and wonderful relief.

Air is your body's first food.
Take in as much of it as you can!

Watch a baby breathe when he or she is asleep. You'll see how the body is supposed to breathe. Watch how the entire rib cage moves easily and completely. It moves up and down and side to side. That's showing you that the lungs are filling up completely and easily. The chest, belly, and back muscles are soft and elastic. Nothing is restricted. The breath is full.

You can do this while you're awake.

1. First, relax your body. Sit or stand with your body naturally upright and relaxed. Keep your spine long and allow your shoulders and rib cage to relax and drop down toward the low belly. Let your chest relax; let the abdominal muscles relax. Let the buttocks and the lower belly relax.

2. Now take a slow breath and allow your abdomen to expand somewhat with the breath. Inhale and exhale as slowly and evenly as you can. Breathe in this way for a few cycles, just allowing your breath to move down into the lower portions of your rib cage. If you feel that your belly or your chest are tight, try to relax them. If your chest or shoulders rise up, let them relax and drop down. Keep your breath slow and deep.

3. Now inhale deeply. Allow your rib cage to relax. As your muscles relax you'll feel as if your body is filling like a balloon—first your belly will fill, then your chest. Your sides will expand and so will your back. This will happen naturally in the relaxed body. In fact, if you watch a person breathe when asleep, you will note exactly this body motion when he or she breathes. It is similar to a container being filled: first the lower portion fills, then the upper portion fills.

4. Now exhale. Let your body relax and you'll see that the upper part of your chest will deflate first, then the lower portion will follow. It's just like a balloon. It deflates evenly and slowly.

5. Try to continue to breathe like this, fully and completely, paying attention to the pitfalls: the shoulders may want to rise up; the abdominal muscles may tighten. Try to keep them relaxed. If you feel as though you're "running out of breath," stop. Breathe normally for a couple of minutes and try again.

Practice this in front of a mirror at first. What you see may surprise you. You may feel as though your body is inflating fully but you might see that only your chest is rising. As you correct yourself, you'll get better and better at this full-body breathing. Practice is essential.

Breathing properly while you are at rest is the first step to retraining the body to breathe properly while you are engaged in activities: sitting at your computer, relaxing at dinner, or practicing your sport. When you have begun to breathe well you will start to notice that your stress levels can be reduced by taking a few deep breaths and allowing your muscles to release. Relaxed muscles move well. There will be a reduced tendency toward muscular injury. Your respiratory capacity will increase, allowing your physical endurance to increase. Your cells will be receiving increased levels of oxygen and all your bodily processes will proceed more efficiently.

You'll feel better. Give it a try.

Enjoy a low-fat, high-fiber diet filled with fresh fruits and vegetables and purified water.
We've all heard the phrase "You are what you eat," but few of us actually consider what this really means. Its meaning is quite direct. Our body is *literally* comprised of the components we bring to it when we eat. Before you eat something, think about what ingredients it contains and what those ingredients bring to your body.

Foods to enjoy
Low-fat proteins: fish, chicken, turkey, lean cuts of beef and lamb, eggs, beans, nuts and seeds
Grains and whole-grain products: oats, brown rice, barley, buckwheat
Fresh fruits and vegetables: organic fruits and vegetables are highly recommended when available

Low-fat dairy products

Olive oil

Foods rich in omega-3 fatty acids, such as wild cold-water fish and flax seed

Foods to limit or eliminate

(The rule of thumb: If you can't pronounce it, think twice about eating it!)

foods containing preservatives, additives, chemicals

fruits and vegetables grown with pesticides

meats from animals raised with hormones and antibiotics

artificial sweeteners

foods containing high percentages of processed sugars and flours (including certain breads, cookies, cakes, and snack foods containing primarily processed ingredients)

hydrogenated oils; trans fats; saturated fats

Eat and drink properly (and enough) for your sport.

Try to eat and drink in sync with your workouts. Think about the demands that your sport is placing on your body and try to consider what and when you eat in order to meet those demands.

1. Consume a light meal of nutrient-dense carbohydrates, such as whole grains, beans, or legumes, several hours prior to activity. This will help you make it through the workout with energy and vitality.

2. Proteins assist with muscle repair; therefore, it is important to consume a protein meal after dancing or working out. After a class or a workout try a snack that is half-protein and half-carbohydrate, such as a peanut butter sandwich. Proteins at a dinner meal will help repair tissue and prepare you for the next day's work.

3. Drink plenty of purified water.

   Thirst is not necessarily a measure of need. This is particularly true during exercise. My son's high school wrestling coach told the boys that "urine should be clear and copious." Perhaps it shouldn't *always* be clear and copious, but certainly once a day your urine should be clear. Dark yellow urine is urine that is highly concentrated, possibly indicating dehydration. Drink water throughout the day and pay attention to the color of your urine. It's not a good idea to concentrate your fluid intake into just a few hours of the day, so spread out your fluid intake throughout the day and early evening. If the need to urinate frequently wakens you from sleep, reduce your fluid intake after dinner; balance that with increased fluid intake during the day.

Generally speaking, approximately 64 ounces of fluid from most sources taken throughout the day should be sufficient. However, if you are engaging in vigorous exercise the following hydration guide is recommended:

Within two hours before vigorous activity, drink 16 to 24 ounces (two to three 8-ounce glasses) of water. (Hikers, particularly those who are hiking in hot or dry climates, are often advised to "camel up"—to drink as much as one quart of water within an hour of beginning their hike.)

During activity, 4 to 8 ounces of water should be consumed approximately every thirty minutes.

To increase fluid absorption, drink water that is approximately 40 to 50 degrees Farenheit in temperature. This will increase the rate at which the stomach empties, and the water will become absorbed into the tissues faster than warmer water.

4. Consume sufficient water to replace the fluids that you've lost during a day's workout. With a heavy workout you should consume more than 64 ounces daily.

5. Try to avoid sugared drinks. They will stay in your stomach longer than water and will thus hinder rehydration. They will also have an adverse effect on your blood sugar balance. You will trade in an immediate burst of energy for an energy deficit shortly thereafter.

6. Coffee dehydrates the kidneys and produces an artificial energy boost. Try to avoid drinking more than one or two cups daily.

7. Alcohol dehydrates the kidneys. If you do consume alcoholic beverages, drink only in moderation and balance the dehydration that results from alcohol consumption by increasing your water consumption.

8. Snack on nutrient-dense, low-sugar foods such as fruits, nuts, seeds, low-fat cheeses, and low-fat yogurt.

9. Don't skip meals. Your body *needs* fuel to meet the high-energy demands that vigorous activity places on us.

Rest and sleep in the name of muscle repair.

Sleep is so important; it rejuvenates. So is rest, and by rest I mean allowing the muscles that you use for your sport to relax and repair themselves. Let your muscles heal between workouts. Muscle repair requires time. In the best of circumstances, twenty-four to thirty-six hours should pass between heavy workouts or classes to allow muscle repair. Deep repair takes place during sleep; make sure that you are getting enough. For the average adult, seven hours' sleep is generally adequate.

If you find that your body is fatigued, or you are having a particularly difficult time physically, respect the moment and the need. Let your body rest. Don't push yourself too hard. Other days will come in which you will be functioning at a higher level. We all have cycles. Accept all parts of those cycles—the highs and the lows. Pushing yourself during a cycle of fatigue is one of the most common causes of musculoskeletal injury during exercise.

As adult athletes we may not be able to perform seven days a week, like we did when we were kids. Our bodies might not want us to play ball all day Saturday *and* Sunday, or to play three sets of tennis followed by eighteen holes of golf on a day off. If you recognize this truth and act on it before your body alerts you to the reality by getting hurt, you will be much happier in the long run. Take a day off in between workouts. Let your muscles rest and heal. Practice one sport a day rather than several. Take one dance or martial arts class, or two classes at most in a given day, and let your body rest for the remainder of the day. If you are a gardener, which involves very hard work, don't do heavy planting or spring clean-up in the morning and expect to be able to function well physically in the afternoon. Pace yourself. This is very important.

Give an injury time to heal.

Nobody likes to admit it, but all athletes at some time or another become injured. It is a sad truth that as we get older our bodies are more easily injured, and those injuries tend to be worse than when we were younger and tend not to heal as rapidly as they did then. You can see this even in your daily life. In your twenties when you had a cold it went through your system in three to five days. In our mature years a cold can take five to seven days to make its way through the body. Bruises need more time to heal completely; the body is not recovering as swiftly as it did years ago.

It follows, then, that if you do injure yourself, whether the injury is related to the activity you love to do or something else, you must let the body heal before you resume your activity. We are often so tempted to work through the pain, but this is never truly successful—especially not once we've reached the magic age of forty. A sprain or muscle strain must heal before you work out again, otherwise the likelihood is that you will reinjure yourself or, worse, produce muscular compensations that will, either immediately or over time, produce physical dysfunction.

So take care of injuries immediately, should they occur. The notion that "it will go away" is generally a hope rather than a reality, particularly in the mature, active years.

If you do become injured, apply RICE—rest, ice, compression, and elevation—within the first twenty-four to forty-eight hours, and with a joint-related injury. Anti-inflammatories to reduce swelling are useful if needed but should not be taken for more than a few days without medical supervision. If you have any doubt as to the severity of an injury, seek medical evaluation.

If you do develop an injury, give yourself ample time to heal before resuming physical activities that stress that muscle group.

The application of moist heat, through the use of a wet heating pad or soaking in a tub of warm water, is very useful in the treatment of sore, restricted musculature.

I'll repeat the truth that we like to hear least of all: taking time off to heal is sometimes necessary. It ultimately allows you to practice your sport with greater frequency over time. Taking time off is difficult to do, but it is the rational thing to do.

Don't use painkillers to mask pain.
We live in an "aspirin society." So many of us want to take a pill and make our physical problems go away. A pill is fast and it's easy. Unfortunately it's also harmful in the long run. One of the purposes of pain is to alert you to a problem in a given area of the body. Pain hampers your ability to use that part of your body. Pain prevents continuous action. When pain is masked the dysfunctional body part is used freely—increased injury often results from the overuse.

Learn to use pain to your advantage. When a part of the body hurts, it requires attention. That attention might be as little as rest or as much as a visit to a health care practitioner. Whatever your body may need, don't mask the pain; don't pretend it isn't there. Take care of the problem instead. Your body will benefit in the long run.

Respect your limitations.

Natural athletes are few and far between, and most of the time they are the ones who have become professionals. Physical shape and form, inherent abilities, and age all affect our ability to perform. Understand what your capabilities and limitations are: develop your capabilities and respect your limitations. When you can recognize what your limitations are you can accept them and accept what you can and cannot do in your sport. Sometimes, particularly for the serious amateur athlete, we lose sight of the fact that we are engaging in our sport for fun and good health and we end up pushing our bodies beyond their limits. Worse still, we become upset, disappointed, or frustrated because we find that our bodies will not and cannot perform as well as we'd like. It's so important to remember that we aren't practicing for auditions for a professional league or corps de ballet. We really are doing our sport or our art because it brings us joy: we love the movement, we love the way it feels in our bodies, and we love the camaraderie. Remember who you are and why you are engaging in your sport. By doing so you'll find emotional peace as well as physical pleasure.

**Work regularly with a health care practitioner
who understands the musculature.**

Any athlete will tell you that your muscles will work better if they are worked on. This is important regardless of age, but it is especially important as we move through our mature years. Muscles should be supple and elastic. Daily life, age, stresses, activities all contribute to the physical tension that we experience as our muscles get tighter. Often our emotional tension is both reflected in and is a reflection of our physical tension.

One of the best ways to deal with this inevitable physical tension is to work with someone who is knowledgeable about the muscular system and to work with that practitioner long enough that he or she becomes knowledgeable about *your* muscular system. There are many health care practitioners who are capable of doing trigger point therapy: massage therapists, acupuncturists, physical therapists, osteopaths, and chiropractors to name a few. By having our muscles cared for on a regular basis, be it once a week or once a month or even several times a year, injuries can be prevented because the muscles will be kneaded and released before they become problematic.

Utilizing these guidelines may seem a bit daunting, but most of these suggestions will incorporate themselves into your life if you think about them and recognize their value within the context of your life. The smallest changes often bring the greatest results: a small dietary change can lead to a lifetime of greater health; taking a moment to remember to relax and breathe can change your day by defusing the fight that's about to happen; stretching and using your muscles throughout the day will help to prevent Monday's back pain after a weekend of activity; drinking a bit more purified water can lead to far better functioning of your organs, your systems, and your muscles.

If you don't believe that you can do all of these things, try one and see how you feel. Your body will tell you how you are doing and what it needs. It just might tell you that it would like more of that good stuff.

Good luck. Be well.

Associated Muscles

The body is an integrated whole with complicated patterns of muscular interrelationships. That being the case, sometimes muscles might contribute to pain in a particular area, although their trigger points don't specifically refer pain to that area. I'll call these muscles *associated muscles*. During your treatment of the muscles that are the source of your pain, check these muscles out as well. You might find them sore and restricted. Work on them also; their release will contribute to your complete recovery.

Muscles associated with neck and upper back pain
   sternocleidomastoid, p. 28
Muscles associated with head and face pain
   scalenes, pp. 50, 70, 88
   trapezius, p. 42
Muscles associated with shoulder pain
   levator scapulae, p. 44
   rhomboids, p. 48
   serratus anterior, p. 103
   sternocleidomastoid, p. 28
   trapezius, p. 42
Muscles associated with elbow, arm, and hand pain
   biceps brachii, p. 68
   deltoid, p. 66
   levator scapulae, p. 44
   posterior cervicals (semispinalis capitis and semispinalis cervicis),
      pp. 30, 46
   splenius capitis, p. 31

Helpful Treatment Aids

Those of us who work professionally to care for the muscles use our hands as tools. It is through the hands and fingers that we can "see" what is going on in the body—the hands can identify restrictions and feel release.

Hands and fingers can be trained to develop that strength and sensitivity. For practitioners of massage and myofascial therapies, this is a must. For most everybody else, it is not. And while hand and finger strength is a wonderful tool in and of itself (think of how nice it is to be able to open jars!) some people do not have it.

Trigger point treatment tools help compensate for this. Some such tools you have around your house—tennis balls, squash balls, pencil erasers. The Pressure Positive Company has devised several inexpensive handheld tools that can help you direct pressure into the muscle without straining your hands and fingers. Their website can be accessed at www.pressurepositive.com.

A clear mental image of body structures will contribute to your ability to work on your body. The interested reader is encouraged to evolve that image. The *Anatomy Coloring Book* by Wynn Kapit and Lawrence Elson (Harper and Row, New York, 1977) is readily accessible to the layperson. The sections on muscular anatomy are clear and easy to understand; working these pages will help provide the imagery that your fingers will need to "see" when they feel the muscles.

Physical Examination of the Spine and Extremities by Stanley Hoppenfeld, M.D. (Appleton-Century-Crofts, Norwalk, Connecticut, 1976) is an excellent guide to the palpation of bones, muscles, and other anatomical structures. Form and body movement can be further explored in *Anatomy of Movement* by Blandine Calais-Germain (Eastland Press, Seattle, 1985).

Pain Pattern Index

HEAD AND FACE PAIN

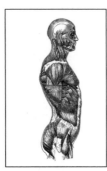

Sternocleidomastoid, p. 28

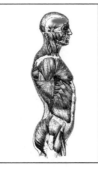

Posterior cervicals (Semispinalis capitis), p. 30

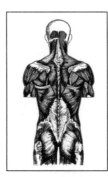

Posterior cervicals (Semispinalis cervicis), p. 30

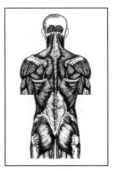

Splenius capitis, p. 31

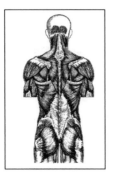

Splenius cervicis, p. 32

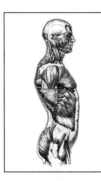

Masseter, p. 33

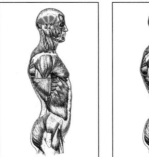

Temporalis, p. 35

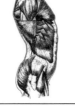

Pterygoids, p. 36

NECK AND UPPER BACK PAIN

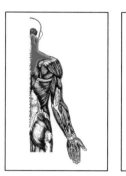
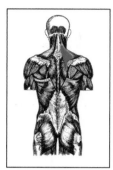
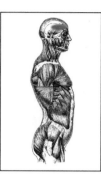

Trapezius, p. 42

Levator scapulae, p. 44

Posterior cervicals
(Semispinalis capitis),
p. 46

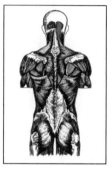
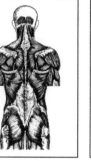
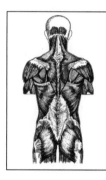

Posterior cervicals
(Semispinalis cervicis),
p. 46

Splenius cervicis, p. 47

Rhomboids, p. 48

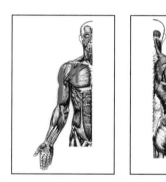

Scalenes, p. 50

SHOULDER PAIN

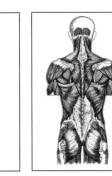
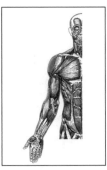

Infraspinatus, p. 56   Teres minor, p. 58   Supraspinatus, p. 59

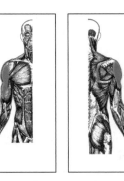
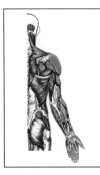
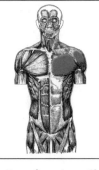
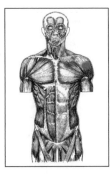

Supraspinatus, p. 59   Subscapularis, p. 60   Pectoralis major, p. 62   Pectoralis minor, p. 64

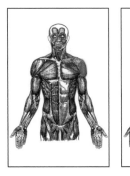
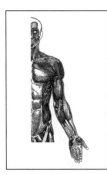
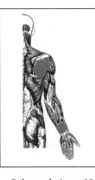

Deltoid, p. 66   Biceps brachii, p. 68   Scalenes, p. 70

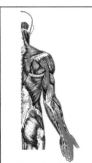
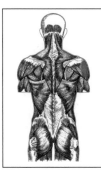
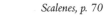

Scalenes, p. 70   Latissimus dorsi, p. 72   Teres major, p. 72

ELBOW, ARM, AND HAND PAIN

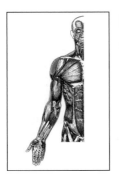

Supraspinatus, p. 78

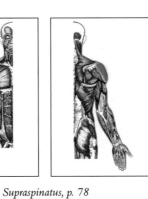

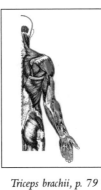

Triceps brachii, p. 79

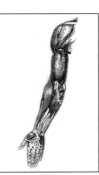

Brachioradialis, p. 80

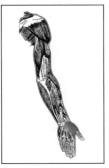

Brachioradialis, p. 80

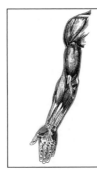

Brachialis, p. 82

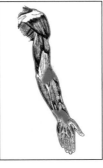

Hand and finger extensors, p. 83

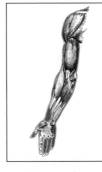

Hand and finger flexors, p. 85

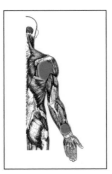

Subscapularis, p. 86

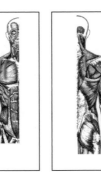

Scalenes, p. 88

TORSO PAIN

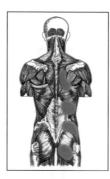

Erector spinae, p. 95

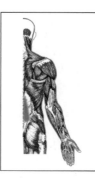

Iliopsoas, p. 97

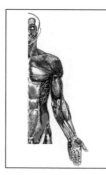

Abdominals (Transversus abdominis, Internal oblique, External oblique), p. 99

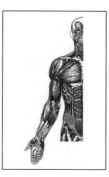

Abdominals (Rectus abdominis), p. 102

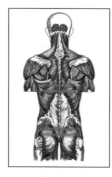

Abdominals (Rectus abdominis), p. 102

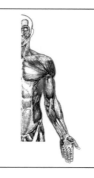

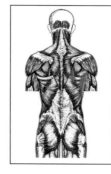

Serratus anterior, p. 103

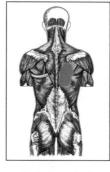

Latissimus dorsi, p. 104

LOW BACK, BUTTOCK, HIP, AND THIGH PAIN

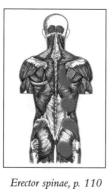

Erector spinae, p. 110

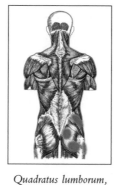

Quadratus lumborum, p. 112

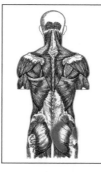

Gluteals (Gluteus maximus), p. 114

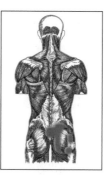

Gluteals (Gluteus medius), p. 117

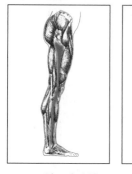

Gluteals (Gluteus minimus), p. 117

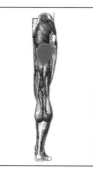

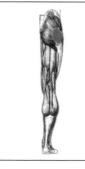

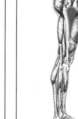

Piriformis, p. 120

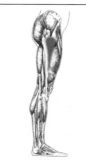

Tensor fasciae latae, p. 122

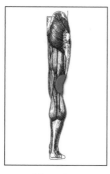

Hamstrings (Biceps femoris), p. 123

Hamstrings (Semitendinosus and Semimembranosus), p. 123

GROIN AND INNER THIGH PAIN

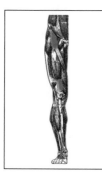

Adductors (Adductor longus and Adductor brevis), p. 130

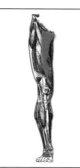

Adductors (Adductor magnus), p. 130

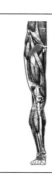

Pectineus, p. 132

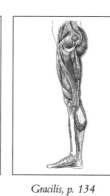

Gracilis, p. 134

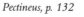

THIGH AND KNEE PAIN

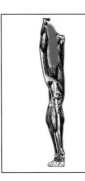

Iliopsoas, p. 140

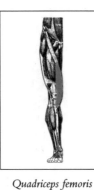

Quadriceps femoris (Vastus medialis), p. 142

Quadriceps femoris (Vastus lateralis), p. 142

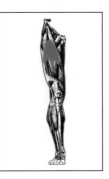

Quadriceps femoris (Vastus intermedius), p. 142

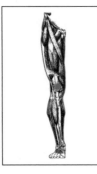

Quadriceps femoris (Rectus femoris), p. 142

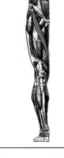

Sartorius, p. 145

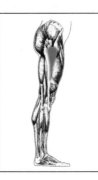

Tensor fasciae latae, p. 146

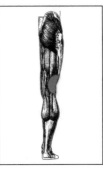

Hamstrings (Biceps femoris), p. 148

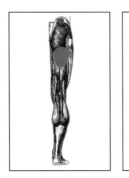

Hamstrings (Semitendinosus and Semimembranosus), p. 148

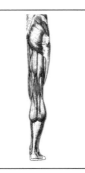

Popliteus, p. 151

LOWER LEG, ANKLE, AND FOOT PAIN

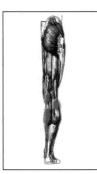

Gastrocnemius, p. 156

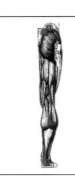

Soleus, p. 158

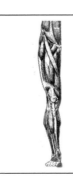

Tibialis anterior, p. 160

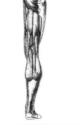

Tibialis posterior, p. 162

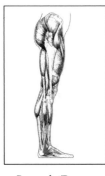

Peroneals (Peroneus longus and Peroneus brevis), p. 163

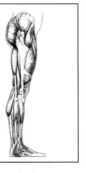

Peroneals (Peroneus tertius), p. 163

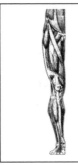

Long extensors of the toes (Extensor digitorum longus), p. 165

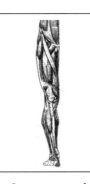

Long extensors of the toes (Extensor hallucis longus), p. 165

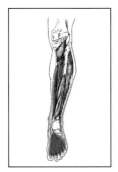

Long flexors of the toes (Flexor digitorum longus), p. 167

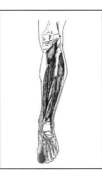

Long flexors of the toes (Flexor hallucis longus), p. 167

Symptom Index

HEAD AND FACE

Blurred vision
    splenius cervicis, 32
Cough (dry)
    sternocleidomastoid, 28
Dizziness
    sternocleidomastoid, 28
Eye redness
    sternocleidomastoid, 28
Headache
    splenius cervicis, 32
    sternocleidomastoid, 28
    temporalis, 35
    trapezius, 42
Hearing loss
    sternocleidomastoid, 28
Imbalance
    sternocleidomastoid, 28
Pain
    ear
        masseter, 33
        sternocleidomastoid, 28
    eye
        splenius cervicis, 32
        sternocleidomastoid, 28
    facial
        masseter, 33
        sternocleidomastoid, 28
        temporalis, 35
    forehead
        semispinalis capitis, 30
        sternocleidomastoid, 28
    head
        base of skull
            trapezius, 42
        side of
            trapezius, 42
        top of
            splenius capitis, 31
            sternocleidomastoid, 28
    jaw
        masseter, 33
        pterygoids, 36
        temporalis, 35
    mouth
        pterygoids, 36
    temple
        semispinalis capitis, 30
        semispinalis cervicis, 30
        sternocleidomastoid, 28
        trapezius, 42
    tooth
        masseter, 33
        temporalis, 35
Reduced range of motion, jaw
    masseter, 33
    pterygoids, 36
Sore throat
    pterygoids, 36
    sternocleidomastoid, 28
Swallowing difficulty
    pterygoids, 36
Tearing
    sternocleidomastoid, 28
Tenderness
    posterior head
        semispinalis capitis, 30
        semispinalis cervicis, 30
    scalp
        sternocleidomastoid, 28

Symptom Index

TORSO

LOW BACK, BUTTOCK, HIP, AND THIGH

GROIN AND INNER THIGH

Bladder pain or difficulties
    (including urinary frequency)
    adductor magnus, 130
    internal oblique, 99
Gynecological difficulties
    (dysmennorhea) or pain
    (menstrual cramping)
    adductor magnus, 130
    rectus abdominis, 102
Pain
    bladder
        adductor magnus, 130
        internal oblique, 99
    groin
        adductor brevis, 130
        adductor longus, 130
        adductor magnus, 130
        external oblique, 99
        iliopsoas, 97, 140
        internal oblique, 99
        pectineus, 132
        transversus abdominis, 99
    inner thigh
        adductor brevis, 130
        adductor longus/
            adductor magnus, 130
        gracilis, 134
    menstrual
        adductor magnus, 130
        rectus abdominis, 102
    pelvic
        adductor magnus, 130
    pubic bone
        adductor magnus, 130
    rectal
        adductor magnus, 130
    vaginal
        adductor magnus, 130
Pelvic inflammatory disease
    adductor magnus, 130

THIGH AND KNEE

Difficulty with movement
    ascending stairs
        quadriceps (vastus inter-
            medius), 142

buckling of the knee
    quadriceps (vastus medialis),
        142
descending stairs
    quadriceps (rectus femoris),
        142
inability to straighten the knee
    popliteus, 151
    quadriceps (vastus inter-
        medius), 142
knee stiffness
    adductor brevis, 130
    adductor longus, 130
rising from a seated position
    erector spinae, 95, 110
    gluteus minimus, 117
    hamstrings (semimem-
        branosus), 148
    quadriceps (vastus inter-
        medius), 142
side lying
    gluteus medius, 117
    gluteus minimus, 117
    quadriceps (vastus lateralis),
        142
    tensor fasciae latae, 146
sitting
    gluteus maximus, 114
    gluteus medius, 117
    hamstrings (biceps femoris,
        semimembranosus, semi-
        tendinosus), 123, 148
    piriformis, 120
    tensor fascie latae, 146
straightening the knee
    popliteus, 151
    quadriceps (vastus inter-
        medius), 142
walking
    gluteus medius, 117
    hamstrings (biceps femoris,
        semimembranosus, semi-
        tendinosus), 123, 148
    piriformis, 120
    quadratus lumborum, 112
    quadriceps (vastus lateralis),
        142
    tensor fasciae latae, 146

Pain

  knee

    back (posterior) of knee

      gastrocnemius, 156

      gluteus minimus, 117

      hamstrings (biceps femoris, semimembranosus, semi-tendinosus), 148

      popliteus, 151

      quadriceps (vastus lateralis), 142

    front (anterior) of knee

      adductor brevis, 130

      adductor longus, 130

      quadriceps (vastus medialis), 142

      quadriceps (rectus femoris), 142

    inside (medial) knee

      adductor brevis, 130

      adductor longus, 130

      hamstrings (semimembranosus, semitendinosus), 148

      quadriceps (vastus medialis), 142

    outside (lateral) knee

      gluteus minimus, 117

      hamstrings (biceps femoris), 148

      quadriceps (vastus lateralis), 142

  hip

    gluteus maximus, 114

    gluteus minimus, 117

    piriformis, 120

    quadratus lumborum, 112

    quadriceps (vastus lateralis), 142

    tensor fasciae latae, 146

  iliac crest

    erector spinae, 95, 110

    gluteus medius, 117

    quadratus lumborum, 112

    quadriceps (vastus lateralis), 142

  thigh

    back (posterior)

      gluteus maximus, 114

      gluteus medius, 117

      gluteus minimus, 117

      hamstrings (biceps femoris, semimembranosus, semi-tendinosus), 148

      piriformis, 120

    front (anterior) of thigh

      iliopsoas, 140

      quadriceps (vastus intermedius), 142

      sartorius, 145

    inside (medial) of thigh

      adductor brevis, 130

      adductor longus, 130

      adductor magnus, 130

      gracilis, 134

      hamstrings (semimembranosus, semitendinosus), 148

      quadriceps (vastus medialis), 142

      sartorius, 145

    outside (lateral side) of thigh

      gluteus minimus, 117

      hamstrings (biceps femoris), 148

      quadriceps (vastus intermedius, vastus lateralis), 142

      tensor fasciae latae, 146

Reduced range of motion

  abduction

    adductor brevis, 130

    adductor longus, 130

  external rotation

    adductor brevis, 130

    adductor longus, 130

LOWER LEG, ANKLE, AND FOOT

Achilles tendinitis

  soleus, 158

Ankle sprain
    peroneus brevis, 163
    peroneus longus, 163
    peroneus tertius, 163
Ankle weakness/instability
    peroneus brevis, 163
    peroneus longus, 163
    peroneus tertius, 163
    tibialis anterior, 160
Cramps
    calf
        gastrocnemius, 156
    foot
        extensor digitorum longus, 165
Difficulty with movement
    dorsiflexion
        soleus, 158
    standing
        flexor digitorum longus, 167
        flexor hallucis longus, 167
    straightening the knee
        gastrocnemius, 156
    walking
        tibialis anterior, 160
        tibialis posterior, 162
    walking down stairs
        soleus, 158
    walking up hills
        soleus, 158
Pain
    Achilles tendon
        soleus, 158
        tibialis posterior, 162
    ankle
        extensor digitorum longus, 165
        gastrocnemius, 156
        gluteus minimus, 117
        peroneus brevis, 163
        peroneus longus, 163
        peroneus tertius, 163
        tibialis anterior, 160
    arch
        tibialis posterior, 162
    calf
        gastrocnemius, 156
        gluteus minimus, 117

    hamstrings (semimembranosus,
        semitendinosus), 123, 148
    soleus, 158
    tibialis posterior, 162
    foot
        extensor digitorum longus, 165
        flexor digitorum longus, 167
        gastrocnemius, 156
        gluteus minimus, 117
    heel
        soleus, 158
    leg
        inside (medial)
            adductor brevis, 130
        outside (lateral)
            gluteus minimus, 117
            tibialis anterior, 160
        shin
            tibialis anterior, 160
        sole
            flexor digitorum longus,
                167
            flexor hallucis longus, 167
            tibialis posterior, 162
        toes
            extensor digitorum longus,
                165
            extensor hallucis longus, 165
            flexor digitorum longus,
                167
            flexor hallucis longus, 167
            tibialis anterior, 160
            tibialis posterior, 162
Tenderness
    Achilles tendon
        soleus, 158
    heel
        soleus, 158
Toes
    clawtoes
        flexor digitorum longus, 167
    hammertoes
        extensor digitorum longus, 165
        flexor digitorum longus, 167